Don't Worry About It

Health Advice You Can Ignore

Connie Leas

Table of Contents

Author's Note

I started writing this book at age eighty-five. Because I'm still alive and well, I think I have a certain credibility when it comes to health-related choices. (This is not to say my health is perfect. I think there's no such thing.) I don't have annual checkups and take no prescription medicines. I see a doctor if I can't fix a problem on my own. But I'm not foolhardy: I got my Covid shots as soon as they were available.

I don't worry about my blood pressure, cholesterol, or germs. I'm unconcerned about how much sleep I get, water I drink, or saturated fats I eat. I wrote this book because I think people worry unnecessarily about such things. We have enough to worry about.

I began collecting the material for this book in 2015 when I launched my blog, "Keeping the Doctor Away" (medfreehealth.blogspot.com). The information comes from trusted sources, such as *The New York Times*, as well as from medical journals. Where the scientific experts disagree, I choose the side that makes the most sense to me.

Connie Leas
September, 2022

1. The Annual Checkup

I had my last annual checkup in 2002. On that occasion my doctor informed me that my cholesterol was high. I'm not worried about mine and don't believe in taking cholesterol-lowering drugs (see Chapter 4). Because I didn't want to argue, I simply never went back for another checkup. It turns out, eliminating annual checkups is probably a wise decision for most of us.

You probably get annual checkups because you think they might prevent you from becoming ill. I used to think that also. But I have since learned that reputable medical organizations agree with my stance. For example, one of the recommendations of the Society of General Internal Medicine's "Choosing Wisely" campaign is *"Don't perform routine general health checks for asymptomatic adults"* [my italics]—asymptomatic meaning you feel fine. Regularly scheduled general health checks, according to this group of doctors, "have not shown to be effective in reducing morbidity, mortality or hospitalization, while *creating a potential for harm from unnecessary testing"* [my italics again]. This conclusion was the result of studies that included nine trials of 155,899 patients.

Other health experts agree. For example, Dr. Ateev Mehrotra, a primary care physician and professor of health policy at Harvard Medical School says, "Patients should really only go to the doctor if something is wrong, or if it's time to have an important preventive test like a colonoscopy." Plus, he says, annual physicals are a waste of money, costing us about $10 billion a year, which is more than we spend on breast cancer. Dr. Ezekiel J. Emanuel, oncologist, and a vice provost at the University of Pennsylvania, says, "from a health perspective, the annual physical exam is basically worthless."

The United States Preventive Services Task Force — an independent group of experts making evidence-based recommendations about the use of preventive services — does not recommend routine annual health checkups. Likewise, the Canadian guidelines have recommended *against* these exams since 1979.

The Cochrane Collaboration, an international group of medical researchers, concluded that annual physicals do not reduce mortality overall, and, specifically, not from deaths caused by cancer or heart disease. To reach this conclusion they examined the records of 182,000 people from 1963 to 1999. This organization, which is made up of 37,000 contributors from more than 130 countries, reviews the world's biomedical research to produce credible health information free from commercial sponsorship. In other words, they study the best evidence from research to determine whether treatments actually work.

By the way, the Cochrane Collaboration is named after Archibald Cochrane who was a prisoner of war in Germany during the Second World War. He was put in charge of overseeing the health of 20,000 fellow prisoners who suffered from diarrhea, typhoid, diphtheria, and other infections. Except for aspirin and antacids, he had no medicine to treat these prisoners. He expected hundreds to die. But in his six months at the camp, only four prisoners died, three of whom had been shot by their captors. When he returned to Britain, he began to question many of the standard medical practices—such as bed rest after a heart attack—that were later shown to be ineffective. He was also instrumental in calling for more randomized trials to test the efficacy of medical treatments.

You can go to the Cochrane Collaboration website and look up the results of their studies. For example, I randomly chose "Acupuncture for tension-type headache" and got the following report: "The available evidence suggests that a course of acupuncture consisting of at least six treatment sessions can be a valuable option for people with frequent tension-type headaches." To come to this conclusion, they "reviewed 12 trials with 2349 adults, published up to January 2016." It's a good site for looking up medical treatments.

Dr. Michael Rothberg, a primary care physician and health researcher at the Cleveland Clinic, tries to avoid giving physicals. "I generally don't like to frighten people, and I don't like to give them diseases they don't have. If you get near doctors, they'll start to look for things and order tests because that's what doctors do." Dr. Gilbert Welch, author of *Overdiagnosed*, tells us that American medicine is "expanding relentlessly." A major reason for this expansion is an increasing tendency to make diagnoses. As Dr. Rothberg said, a doctor will "look for things and order tests." In fact, Welch calls our current situation an "epidemic of diagnoses." Conventional wisdom would have you believe that finding problems early saves lives—that you can fix small problems before they become big problems. But these "small problems" are likely to be little abnormalities that would never bother us. And more diagnoses lead to excessive treatment for problems that aren't bothersome at all. ("Over-diagnosis" by the way, refers to diagnosing a supposed condition that will never cause symptoms or death.)

Cardiologist Sandeep Juahar maintains that a substantial amount of health care in America is wasteful. Many tests and treatments are unnecessary and potentially harmful. He cites a number of reasons: doctors practicing "defensive" medicine to avoid lawsuits; a reluctance to accept diagnostic uncertainty, which leads to more tests; exorbitant prices; lack of consensus about which treatments are effective; and the pervasive belief that newer, more expensive technology is always better. In fact, he says, "perhaps Americans don't require the volume of care that their doctors are used to providing. ...More care doesn't always result in better outcomes."

Studies suggest that up to 20 percent of surgeries in some specialties are unnecessary. Doctors themselves admit that 15 to 30 percent of health care is probably unnecessary. In a survey of 2,106 physicians, about sixty percent reported that patients demanded unnecessary treatment and that 20.6 percent of all medical care was unnecessary, including 22 percent of prescriptions, 24.9 percent of tests, and 11.1 percent of procedures. For example, they believe that a quarter of all spine surgeries may not be necessary. Ditto for half of all stents placed in arteries.

A list of well-regarded medical societies, such as the Society of General Internal Medicine and the American Academy of Neurology produce lists of procedures to avoid. You can see these lists at choosingwisely.org. The lists run to more than 65 pages!

Americans spend more than $2.5 trillion on health. Are we getting our money's worth? Hardly. The United States ranks forty-fifth in life expectancy, behind Bosnia and Jordan. We also rank near last in infant mortality compared with other developed countries. And, according to the Commonwealth Fund, a health care research group, we rank *last* place in health care quality, access, and efficiency when compared to major industrialized countries.

Clearly, over-testing, over-medicating and over-diagnosing people—turning them into patients in need of treatment—has not improved the health of Americans. The Department of Health and Human Service's program, called "Healthy People 2010," reported that between 1999 to 2002 healthy life expectancy (the number of years Americans live free of disease) had *fallen* from 48.7 to 47.5 years. People have gotten sicker. On top of that, unnecessary tests add an estimated $150 billion each year to the health care budget.

It's true that the average lifespan of people in the United States has, since 1900, lengthened by greater than 30 years. But, according to the U.S. Centers for Disease Control, most of this gain (25 years) is attributable to advances in public health, such as sanitation. Of the remaining five years' increased longevity, 18 or 19 months is attributable to preventive care, such as immunizations; and the final 44 to 45 months is attributable to medical care for illness, such as heart attacks, trauma, and cancer treatment. Remember, this longevity increase is for the entire 20th century.

At the time of this writing, federal health researchers reported that life expectancy dropped from 79 in 2109 to 76 in 2021—the sharpest decline in nearly 100 years. While Covid has driven most of the decline, accidental deaths and drug overdoses also contributed, as did deaths from heart disease, chronic liver disease and cirrhosis. Dr. Steven Woolf, director emeritus of the Center on Society and Health at Virginia Commonwealth University, characterized this drop as 'historic." While other high-income countries were also hard hit in 2020, most had begun to recover in 2021. The U.S. had not. "None of them experienced a continuing fall in life expectancy like the U.S. did, and a good number of them saw life expectancy start inching back to normal."

As far as I can tell, skipping annual checkups hasn't affected my health. I seek medical attention if I have a problem I can't fix myself. Otherwise, I save Medicare some money by skipping the checkups and save myself the annoyance of dealing with the medical establishment and undergoing unnecessary tests.

2. Unnecessary Medical Tests

Tests are a significant source of revenue for medical institutions. As Elisabeth Rosenthal writes in *The New York Times*, "Testing has become to the United States' medical system what liquor is to the hospitality industry: a profit center with large and often arbitrary markups." As you might imagine, medical tests are often performed without a legitimate need for them. What's more, they can make matters worse.

In his book *Overdiagnosis,* Dr. Welch tells the following story: As part of her annual checkup, a sixty-five-year-old woman was screened for osteoporosis. She was told that her bone density was a little below average for her age and that she was at risk for bone fractures. (She did not actually have osteoporosis.) Her doctor started her on hormone replacement therapy until it was learned that such therapy increased the risk of heart attack and stroke as well as breast cancer. She was put on a different medication and developed a terrible pain when swallowing. As a result, she was sent to a gastroenterologist who performed an endoscopy and found that she had severe inflammation and ulcers in her esophagus—a known side effect of the drug she had been taking. She was switched to another medicine and the problem with her esophagus went away, but she developed a painful rash and was referred to a dermatologist who suggested she stop the medication. The rash went away, but treatment continued.

Next, she was referred to an endocrinologist who did a thorough evaluation of all her glands and hormones, including a careful physical exam of her thyroid gland, on which the doctor thought he felt a lump. As a result, she was sent to a radiologist, who did an ultrasound exam of her thyroid and found three lumps. To check for cancer of her thyroid, the doctor stuck needles in all the lumps to remove some cells. Under the microscope, the pathologist thought some of the cells looked suspicious and that perhaps her thyroid should be removed. She was referred to a surgeon. Luckily for her, the surgeon put a stop to the whole business, knowing that nearly all adults have some evidence of thyroid cancer. The woman, who was fine before the disastrous bone density screening, is again fine.

The following pages describe some questionable screening procedures:

Screening for thyroid cancer: Unnecessary screening for thyroid cancer is another example of over-testing and over-diagnosis. Supposedly, in the United States, thyroid cancer rates have more than doubled since 1994. But cancer experts agree that cases of thyroid cancer have not actually increased; they have simply been over-diagnosed, which is the case in South Korea. In 1999, a government-funded national cancer screening program in South Korea led to the widespread use of ultrasound to screen for thyroid cancer in people without any symptoms. This program led to an "epidemic" of thyroid cancer in South Korea. But, as reported in the *BMJ*—a journal published by the British Medical Association—this increase of cancer is "due to an increase in the detection of small tumours, most likely as a result of overdetection. Concerted efforts are needed at a national level to reduce unnecessary thyroid ultrasound examinations in the asymptomatic general population."

In the United States and Europe, where screening for thyroid cancer is not a common practice, small tumors may be discovered when patients are scanned for other conditions, such as when performing ultrasound exams of the carotid artery. When performing such screens, doctors are in fact finding very tiny tumors—tumors that are non-aggressive and unlikely to amount to anything. In fact, autopsies have revealed that as many as a third of all people were found to have thyroid cancers that were never a problem. But here's the thing: even though more tumors are being detected, the death rate from thyroid cancer has remained both low and steady. If early detection were saving lives, death rates should have come down. They have not. Making matters worse, unnecessary screening for thyroid cancer has led to some aggressive and unnecessary surgical procedures—some of which have been disastrous ("Oops. Cut a vocal cord"). This happened in two percent of the surgeries in South Korea. Many in the medical profession counsel leaving a newly-detected tumor alone. However, they're finding it a tough sell. Fearful patients are reluctant to take the "do nothing" advice. As for the doctors, one said, "In the US, we have a fear that if we miss a cancer, the patient will sue."

Mammograms: I've had one or two mammograms. The last one was in 2008. I don't remember why I quit having them, but I'm glad I did quit. Statistically, they've proven to be useless and can be damaging. No recent study has ever shown that mammograms prolonged the lives of American women. Although mammograms save some lives, mammograms haven't had an impact on overall mortality. That is, despite three decades of widespread mammography in the United States, the breast cancer rate is unchanged. Breast cancer screening lowers breast cancer mortality on the order of one person per one thousand over ten years--essentially an insignificant number. As one breast cancer surgeon said, "If mammography was a treatment, we'd never do it. The effect is too small."

In a ten-year Canadian study of 600,000 women in which half were being screened and half were not, researchers found that the mammogram group was just as likely to die as the non-mammogram group. So why bother? In Denmark, a 17-year study of both screened and unscreened women found no difference in incidence between the two groups. But among those who were screened, they found substantial overdiagnosis — that is, detection of tumors that would not become cancers needing treatment. Dr. Karsten Juhl Jorgenson, deputy director of the Nordic Cochrane Center, notes that "Some types of screening are a good idea — colorectal, for example. But breast cancer has a biology that doesn't lend itself to screening. Healthy women get a breast cancer diagnosis, and this has serious psychological consequences and well-known physical harms from unnecessary treatment. We're really doing more harm than good." In Switzerland, the Swiss Medical Board has suggested the screening be halted.

Screenings find cancers, labeled "stage 0," that would never develop into anything serious. This kind of "cancer" is called D.C.I.S., which stands for ductal carcinoma in situ. (Dr. Laura J. Esserman, a breast cancer surgeon at the University of California, San Francisco, believes that the word "carcinoma" should be removed from this diagnosis.) It's a small pile-up of abnormal cells in the lining of the milk duct. You can't feel a lump, but the cell cluster can be seen in a mammogram. Every year about 60,000 American women are diagnosed with this Stage 0 breast cancer. As a result, nearly every one of these women undergoes either a lumpectomy or a mastectomy—often a double mastectomy. A new study reported in the *Journal of the American Medical Association* (JAMA) has shown that most of these painful and deforming surgeries are unnecessary and make no difference in the patients' outcomes. To arrive at this conclusion, the study analyzed data from 100,000 patients over 20 years. Even though 60,000 cases of D.C.I.S. are now being found each year, the incidence of invasive breast cancer has not dropped. It remains at about 240,000 cases a year. Patients who had been surgically treated for D.C.I.S. had about the same likelihood of dying of breast cancer as women in the general population—about 3.3 percent. Those who died did so despite the treatment, not for lack of it. Dr. Steven Narod, director of the Familial Breast Cancer Research Unit, Women's College Research Institute (Canada), says "I think the best way to treat D.C.I.S. is to do nothing."

The problem with over-diagnosing breast cancer is that it leads to more testing: another mammogram, an ultrasound, an MRI, a biopsy. Research has shown that the psychological effects of false alarms, such as stress and anxiety, often persist for three years. For every 1,000 women screened every two years, most will have a false-positive mammogram during the next ten years, 146 will have an unnecessary biopsy, seven will have a fatal case of breast cancer prevented, and 19 will be diagnosed with a cancer that never would have killed them. Among the 19 per 1000 who are over-diagnosed, 99 percent will have surgery, 70 percent radiation therapy, 70 percent hormone therapy, and 25 percent chemotherapy—all without benefit.

Scientists have no way of knowing who will benefit by screening. You might reasonably choose to have mammograms on the off chance that you might be one of the seven out of a thousand who has her life saved by screening, but also recognizing that you might be one of the nineteen who will undergo unnecessary treatment.

Or, like me, you could skip the whole business. I don't worry about it.

Prostate screenings: There's a big debate over the value of PSA testing, which refers to tests for a prostate-specific antigen, a protein produced by cells in the prostate gland. The antigen is present in small quantities in the blood of normal men and is often elevated in men with prostate cancer. But it is also elevated because of other causes, such as an infection or benign prostatic hyperplasia, a condition that causes an enlarged prostate but is not cancer.

The annual bill for PSA screening is at least $3 billion, much of it paid for by Medicare and the Veterans Administration. The most outspoken critic of the tests is Dr. Richard J. Ablin, who discovered the prostate-specific antigen. He says, "testing should absolutely not be deployed to screen the entire population of men over the age of 50." He believes that the test is still used because "drug companies continue peddling the tests and advocacy groups push prostate cancer awareness by encouraging men to get screened."

In fact, prostate screening is now out of favor. In 2012, the U.S. Preventive Services Task Force recommended against routine screening, having found that the benefits do not outweigh the risks, which include a high rate of false positives. Men with false positives undergo painful biopsies that find no cancer. Plus, the biopsies themselves cause problems—such as fever, infection, bleeding, and urinary problems—in one out of every three men. And even when a biopsy finds cancer, there is no way to know if it's aggressive or slow growing, in which case it would never be a problem.

Autopsy studies have shown that approximately one third of men aged 40 to 60 years have the slow-growing prostate cancer; for men older than 85, the proportion is three-fourths. In other words, these men die *with* the cancer, not because of it. One important study found no difference in death rates between men who had surgery or radiation and those who were actively monitored and who were treated only if the cancer progressed. (Active monitoring involves regular exams of the prostate, periodic biopsies, and PSA tests that may indicate the disease is worsening.) Also, death rates were low: only about one percent of patients died ten years after the diagnosis. The decision to surgically remove the prostate is not trivial: risks include death, urinary incontinence, impotence, and bowel dysfunction.

I'm glad I don't have to worry about that.

Bone density screening: In 1993, a World Health Organization study group established clear-cut definitions of osteoporosis and osteopenia. (Osteoporosis is a thinning of the bones due to depletion of calcium and bone proteins; osteopenia is bone density that is below "normal.") Their definitions are based on the bone density of healthy young adult women. Thus, if your bone density doesn't measure up to that of a young person, you either have osteopenia or osteoporosis. As it turns out, the WHO study was funded by three drug companies: the Rorer Foundation, Sandoz, and SmithKline Beecham. These companies stood to benefit greatly if bone mineral density testing was adopted into routine medical care—which it has been. Because loss of bone density is a normal part of aging, millions of women use drugs hoping to prevent and treat osteoporosis. They don't want to fall and break a hip.

The most dangerous result of falling for an older person is a hip fracture. But bone density tests identify only a small part of the risk of hip fracture. For women between the ages of 60 and 80 only one-sixth of their risk of fracturing a hip is identified by bone density testing. Just as important are muscle weakness, the side of effects of other drugs, declining vision, and cigarette smoking. On top of that, the osteoporosis drugs don't protect women from hip fractures, which is the primary reason for taking the drugs. One study, for example, showed that the risk of hip fractures actually went up with Fosamax treatment. The reason drugs like Fosamax are ineffective is that they act on only one of the two bone types—the outer, hard cortical layer. They do not add bone to the internal structure called the trabecular bone, which works like a three-dimensional geodesic dome to provide additional strength to the areas of the skeleton most vulnerable to fracture, such as the hips, wrists, and spine. A new class of drugs, such as Evista, is designed to protect bones the same way that natural estrogen does, but without the risk of hormone therapy. However, research shows that in women with osteoporosis, Evista reduces only vertebral fractures, not fractures of the hip or wrist.

The best protection against hip fractures is—you guessed it—exercise. Example: The National Institutes of Health conducted a study of osteoporotic fractures in which they followed 10,000 independently living women aged 65 and older. Over the seven years of the study, women who exercised moderately had 36 percent fewer hip fractures than the least active women. In this case, the reduction of hip fractures among those who exercised was twice that achieved with Fosamax.

I've never had a bone mineral density test and I don't worry about having osteoporosis.

Echocardiograms and angiograms: In the words of Dr. Eric J. Topol, a cardiologist at Scripps Health in San Diego, "At many hospitals, the threshold for ordering an echocardiogram is the presence of a heart." (An echocardiogram is an ultrasound picture of the heart.) For example, one internist required that his patient have an echocardiogram before having elective cataract surgery, a requirement that goes against the recommendation of the echocardiography professional society. That organization specifically advises against ordering the test for preoperative assessment of patients with no history or symptoms of heart disease.

Echocardiograms continue to be an important source of income for many hospitals. The charge for these tests is high and varies from place to place. For example, one patient was billed $1,400 at one location and $5,500 at another. The cost of medical technology equipment is often the excuse for the high prices, but echocardiography equipment, as well as many other technologies, have become cheaper, just as high-definition TVs have. Electrocardiography devices can now be purchased for as little as $5,000.

17

Angiograms are also performed unnecessarily. (Angiograms look for blocked arteries, using a thin tube injected with dye, which makes arteries visible on X-rays.) Every year in the United States, more than a million people get an angiogram, frequently without a sound basis for doing so. The American College of Cardiology sponsored a study of such cases, which consisted of nearly two million angiograms. In analyzing the data, the researchers found no significant artery blockages in 62 percent of the angiograms.

If you have a completely blocked artery, these procedures may be lifesaving. But angiograms are frequently performed as elective procedures on people with no symptoms of heart problems. According to the American Medical Association, 35 percent of the procedures are "inappropriate" and another third are questionable. That's a lot, especially considering that the procedure typically costs around $8,000 and angioplasty costs about $30,000. (An efficient "cath lab" in a hospital can perform around twelve diagnostic angiograms in a day—a big money maker.) Moreover, while major complications are not common, the procedure can cause tears in blood vessel walls and major bleeding.

The thing is, there's no predicting where a heart attack will originate. It could start anywhere where there is plaque, even if the plaque is not obstructing blood flow. A heart attack occurs when a clot breaks off the plaque and blocks the artery. That is, the plaque doesn't cause trouble until a piece of it breaks off. And it doesn't need to come from a big piece of plaque. A study performed in 2011 found that only a third of heart attacks originated in plaques that were blocking at least half of an artery. The remainder began with the rupture of plaques that appeared to be causing no problems. In other words, the area of an artery that is partly blocked by plaque and visible in an angiogram is no more likely to be the site of a heart attack than a more benign-looking section where the plaque is less pronounced.

You will be unhappy to learn that, according to Dr. Gregg W. Stone, a cardiologist at Columbia, "Half the people over 65 have blockages." We just need to get comfortable with that fact. As Dr. Judith Hochman, a cardiologist at NYU Longone Hospital says, "People believe that if they have a blockage, they have to fix it mechanically. It seems logical, but in medicine, many things that seem logical are not true."

In addition to echocardiograms and angiograms, other heart-related tests are available. You can get stress tests, electrocardiograms, and myocardial perfusion imaging. But, unless you have symptoms of heart problems, researchers reporting in *The Annals of Internal Medicine* conclude that these tests have not been shown to improve patient outcomes and can lead to potential harm. The tests commonly produce false positives that lead to further unnecessary testing, and all of them involve extra expense.

I've never had any of these tests.

Imaging overuse—something to worry about: Sometimes scans are needed for diagnostic purposes—but often they're not. The various scan types include X-rays,

MRIs, and CT/CAT scans. X-rays use invisible electromagnetic energy beams to produce images of internal tissues, bones, and organs on film or digital media. An MRI scan uses magnetic fields and computer-generated radio waves to create detailed images of the organs and tissues in your body. Most MRI machines are large, tube-shaped magnets. CT and CAT scans are basically the same thing. They use a combination of X-rays and computer technology to produce detailed images of any part of the body, including bones, muscles, fat, organs and blood vessels. The machine looks like a large donut.

A consortium of professional medical societies, including the American Society of Radiology, is fighting the overuse of imaging, such as performing routine chest X-rays and scans for nonspecific back pain. Between 2000 and 2007, imaging grew faster than any other physician service in the Medicare population. One study determined that 20 to 50 percent of imaging provides no useful information. The problem with too much imaging (besides unnecessary costs) is that it can expose you to excessive radiation and can also lead to over-diagnosis, which is then followed by unnecessary interventions that can do more harm than good.

Scans can also be dangerous. At least two percent of all future cancers in the U.S.—about 29,000 cases and 15,000 deaths per year—are a result of CT scans alone. Dr. Stephen J. Swensen, medical director at the Mayo Clinic says, "If the scan isn't necessary or emits the wrong dose of radiation, the risks far outweigh the benefits." According to the March 2015 issue of *Consumer Reports* magazine,

"Just one CT scan of the abdomen and pelvis equals about 10 millisieverts, more radiation than most residents of Fukushima, Japan, absorbed after the Fukushima Daichi nuclear power plant accident in 2011." Add to that the fact that there are no federal radiation limits for any kind of imaging and no national standards for training or certifying technologists. Apparently, about one-third of the scanners now used across the country won't meet the safety standards that will soon be required by the Centers for Medicare and Medicaid Services.

There may be cause for worry if you had CT scans as a child. Cancers from medical radiation can take anywhere from five to 60 years to develop. Children are particularly vulnerable to the effects of radiation. Those who had a CT scan before the age of five face a 35 percent spike in cancer risk. For every 1,000 children who have an abdominal CT scan, one will develop cancer as a result. A 2012 study that looked at almost 180,000 British children linked CT scans to higher rates of leukemia and brain cancer. Dr. Swensen says, "All too often children are receiving adult-sized doses of radiation, which is many times the amount they need. The dose directly increases the risk of leukemia or a solid tumor. And that's not regulated today." A friend of mine developed cancer of the salivary gland which she suspects (with good evidence) was caused by X-ray treatments for acne she received as a teenager over 50 years ago. The treatment to remove the cancer was horrible.

A memory: When I was a child in the 1940s, the latest technology at the shoe store was an x-ray machine that would show an eerie green image of the bones of your feet.

The machine was a wooden cabinet with shoe-size slots into which you put your feet, shod in the shoes your mother had chosen for you (in my case, always Girl Scout brown oxfords). At the base of the cabinet was a fluoroscope that emitted X-rays. When the salesperson turned on the machine, you could see your bones, which was rather thrilling. Of course, the machines didn't show the soft tissue around the bones. In fact, the machines were useless—just sales gimmicks.

The typical "X-Ray Shoe Fitting Machine" delivered a radiation dose of 13 roentgen, though some were much higher, especially if the lead shielding had been removed to make moving the heavy cabinets around easier. The dose of radiation was relatively harmless for the occasional shoe shopper. But for the children who tested their feet regularly for fun, the machines posed a serious health risk. They were even more dangerous for the store's staff who often spent most of their workdays around the machines, which often leaked radiation into the store. As early as 1950, the radiation hazards of the machines were already recognized, and states began to ban them. A 2007 Wisconsin Medical Journal report linked the use of the machines to basal cell carcinoma of the sole of the foot. (I've had plenty of basal cell cancers, but none on the soles of my feet, at least none that I've noticed.)

Here is what the *Consumer Reports* magazine offers as are the guidelines for making decisions about getting scans or X-rays, beginning with four scans you can usually skip:

- **X-rays for back pain**: Back pain is usually caused by muscle damage and clears up on its own. Unless your doctor suspects a serious underlying problem such as cancer or a spinal infection, or severe nerve damage, an x-ray is not usually needed.

- **Chest x-rays before surgery**: You don't need to be cleared for surgery with an x-ray unless your surgery involves the heart, lungs, or part of the chest.
- **CT scans to screen for lung cancer**: The test is worthwhile only for people at the highest risk of developing lung cancer, which includes current or former smokers between the ages of 55 and 80 who smoked the equivalent of a pack a day for 30 years.
- **CT scans for headaches**: A CT scan for headaches is necessary only if your doctor can't diagnose your problem based on a physical exam, which he or she almost always can. However, if your headache is sudden or explosive or accompanied by fever, seizure or vomiting, a scan is warranted—but not a CT scan, which exposes you to radiation. Get an MRI instead.

As to X-rays on your teeth (the bitewing type), *Consumer Reports* says you need one only every 24 to 36 months, and you can go a decade between full-mouth x-rays. I generally decline them.

Years ago, I had a problem with my knee. It didn't want to bend, and I wanted to figure out what was wrong with it.

I had an MRI, which takes pictures of soft tissue. It showed that I had a "shredded" meniscus, which caused a fluid build-up. It was the fluid that made it difficult (and painful) to bend my knee. I was glad to learn that, but it probably wasn't necessary. As with the MRI of my knee, imaging and other medical tests can be helpful for diagnosing problems. But be choosy. Don't undergo tests if you're feeling fine. One thing often leads to another. Like the woman in the opening story, you could start out with an osteoporosis test and end up being misdiagnosed with thyroid cancer.

3. Blood Pressure

According to current guidelines, I have high blood pressure. The current guidelines define high ("elevated") blood pressure as 120 to 139, for the upper systolic reading, and 80 to 89 for the lower, diastolic reading. Given these guidelines, nearly half of all American adults and nearly 80 percent of those 65 and older will be considered to have high blood pressure and to need medication for it. I ignore the guidelines. In fact, one reason I avoid annual checkups is my unwillingness to have my blood pressure checked at the doctor's office. It's always high.

High blood pressure (hypertension) was the first condition for which doctors began treating people who weren't feeling sick. Prior to the late 20th century, physicians generally prescribed medicines only to patients with symptoms of disease. Now, people with no health complaints are given a diagnosis of hypertension and prescribed treatment based, usually, on unrealistic measurements. Thus, many healthy people who were never destined to develop symptoms or die from hypertension are needlessly treated—and that's a lot of people.

The definition of what constitutes high blood pressure is regularly revised, constantly creeping lower over time. By lowering the definition of what constitutes high blood pressure, you increase the pool of potential patients who are otherwise healthy, a boon for pharmaceutical companies: treatment for hypertension translates into a $40 billion global market in blood pressure medicines.

Not all physicians buy into the guidelines, which are developed by the American College of Cardiology and American Heart Association. For example, one cardiologist, Wake Forest University professor Curt Furberg, doesn't believe it's a good idea to treat someone with a blood pressure of 160 who is otherwise healthy. The same goes for Dr. Malcolm Kendrick, who argues that "almost everything written about treating blood pressure is wrong." He also notes that "raised blood pressure is not a disease. It is not even symptom of a disease; because a raised blood pressure does not cause any symptoms unless it is extremely high." Kendrick also tells us that "… there is almost no correlation between the amount the blood pressure is lowered (at the arm) – and any clinical outcomes. By which I mean that the rate of heart attacks and strokes do not relate to the degree of blood pressure lowering." Dr. Gilbert Welch, a former professor of medicine at the Dartmouth Institute for Health Policy and Clinical Practice, also questions the new guidelines: "a national goal of 130 as measured in actual practice may lead many to be over-medicated--making their blood pressure too low. More medications and lower blood pressures are not always better for everyone."

As I said above, supposedly "normal" blood pressure is less than 120/80. (Blood pressure readings are given in two numbers. The top number—systolic—is the maximum pressure your heart exerts while your heart is beating. The bottom number—diastolic—is the amount of pressure in your arteries between beats.) In fact, nobody really knows the demarcation between "normal" and "abnormal" blood pressure. For one thing, blood pressure varies depending on what you're doing, your stress level, and your surroundings. I remember being stuck in traffic on my way to a doctor appointment and was in a snit when I got there. As I recall, my blood pressure measured around 170 over something. As I said, my blood pressure is always high in a doctor's office—a common phenomenon called the "white coat syndrome."

The U.S. Preventive Services Task Force recommends that patients not be diagnosed as hypertensive based on measurements taken in a medical facility, which means you must measure yourself at home. In the interests of science, I've tested my blood pressure at home and have seen how it varies from time to time—ranging anywhere from 118 to 158. If you have a home BP monitor, you've probably discovered the same thing: your blood pressure is all over the place. Because of the difficulties of measuring the blood pressure, it is estimated that around 25 per cent of people diagnosed as having hypertension do not actually have high blood pressure at all. Which means that they are taking drugs that they do not need.

Of course, extremely high blood pressure, such as 202/117, is abnormally high and should be treated. Blood pressure at these levels will likely cause symptoms, such as severe headache, as was the case for President Franklin D. Roosevelt, whose blood pressure before he died was 300/190. He died of a massive hemorrhage in his brain. In this case, treatment was certainly warranted.

Unnecessary treatment for high blood pressure wouldn't be bad if it weren't for the negative side effects (not to mention cost and bother). For many, blood pressure meds cause dizziness and lightheadedness. Considering that most people over 70 take blood pressure meds, over-treatment can be dangerous. In fact, a study performed in 2014 found that, among older people, the risk of serious injuries from falls was significantly higher for those who took hypertension drugs than for those who did not.

There are quite a variety of blood pressure meds, such as diuretics, beta-blockers, and ACE inhibitors. Some, such as diuretics, make your body get rid of excess salt and water. Others, such as beta-blockers, reduce the heart rate. Still others, such as ACE inhibitors, relax the blood vessels, so the heart doesn't have to work as hard to pump blood throughout the body. Depending on which type of med you're taking, the side effects vary. Some cause fatigue because they slow down the pumping action of the heart and depress the entire central nervous system. The diuretic meds make you pee a lot. In so doing, you deplete important electrolytes, which causes fatigue. Gout is another side effect of diuretics. Because the diuretic type of BP meds increase urination, the amount of fluid in your body is reduced and the remaining fluid is more concentrated, which increases the risk of developing the crystals that cause gout. Similarly, because of the increased loss of water, the diuretic type of BP meds causes the calcium in urine to become more concentrated, which can lead to the formation of calcium (kidney) stones.

In the spring of 2022, I had both knees replaced—one month apart. Of course, at my pre-op appointment I had to undergo the dreaded blood pressure test. Sure enough, it was high—in the mid-190s. The medical personnel were alarmed and insisted that I get clearance from my doctor before I could have the surgeries. At my doctor's office, my blood pressure again approached 200 (systolic). I was given a prescription for meds, a combination of an ACE inhibitor and diuretic. The meds did the trick, allowing me to have the surgery. One morning at home, I was feeling lightheaded and discovered that my blood pressure was only 87. After my surgeries, I quit taking the drugs. In testing myself at home, I've found my numbers to be acceptable, and my doctor has agreed.

Now, for the upside of high blood pressure: it reduces the chance of dementia among the "oldest-old." Two studies have proven this phenomenon. The first is called "The Leiden 85-Plus Study," in which researchers in the Netherlands followed 572 85-year-olds for 3.2 years, measuring their blood pressure, their activities of daily living and their cognitive scores. Their conclusion: "Lower blood pressure during antihypertensive treatment is associated with higher all-cause mortality and accelerated cognitive decline in the oldest-old." Or, as stated in another journal, high blood pressure is "associated with resilience to physical and cognitive decline." Furthermore, subsequent studies of the data have shown that higher systolic blood pressure was "...associated with reduced risk of stroke." So, for my cohort, higher blood pressure protects you from physical and cognitive decline as well as from stroke.

The second study is called "The Leisure World Cohort Study." In 1981, 14,000 residents of a retirement community in California completed lengthy surveys about their health and lifestyles. The surveys were ignored until 2003, when researchers, led by Dr. Claudia Kawas, a neurologist and professor at UC Irvine, discovered this trove of information. In studying the records, her team found that 1,900 of the original survey takers were still alive and in their 90's or older. The researchers tested about 1,600 of this still-alive group for a variety of health indicators. Among other things, their findings revealed that having high blood pressure reduced their chances of dementia. I learned about this from a *60 Minutes* program. Here is a brief excerpt:

60 Minutes announcer: While none of the factors from the original Leisure World study—vitamins, alcohol, caffeine, even exercise—seemed to lower people's risk of getting dementia, the 90-plus study discovered that high blood pressure did.

Claudia Kawas: If you have high blood pressure, it looks like your risk of dementia is lower.

Leslie Stahl: Lower?

Claudia Kawas: Than if you don't—

Leslie Stahl: High blood—

Claudia Kawas: —have high blood pressure.

Lesley Stahl: Wait. High blood pressure, lower risk of dementia?

Claudia Kawas: In a 90-year-old.

4. Cholesterol

I don't worry about my cholesterol. The last time I had it checked was about 20 years ago when it was shown to be 258, a level considered to be high. As far as I'm concerned, all this concern about cholesterol is nonsense. Our livers manufacture cholesterol for a reason: cholesterol is essential to life. For one thing, it constitutes half the dry weight of your cerebral cortex. It's also vital for the proper functioning of many bodily processes. For example, it's essential for producing many important hormones, including testosterone and estrogen; it's used as the raw material in tissue repair; it's an important component of cell membranes; it's used to produce vitamin D; and it facilitates mineral metabolism as well as serotonin uptake in the brain and regulation of blood sugar levels.

Like much else in the natural world, the range of cholesterol levels in a population follows a normal distribution curve—a bell curve—wherein the bulk of the people fall within the average group and fewer people fall within the low and high groups. This is a fundamental and widely used concept of statistical analysis. For example, if you measured the height of the population within a country you would find that a small number of people are very short; most people are average; a small number are very tall. The short, tall, and average-sized people are all normal. The same is true for cholesterol. Some of us naturally have low cholesterol, some naturally have high cholesterol and most of us are somewhere in between. All are normal, but most fall in the 200-250 milligrams per deciliter of blood.

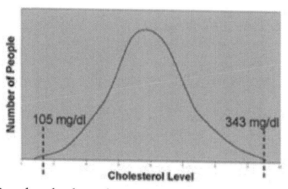

People who have heart disease and people who do not have heart disease fall within this same range. That is, their cholesterol has no bearing on whether they have heart disease, as proven by the Framingham Study, one of the largest studies ever done on cholesterol. Other studies have confirmed this fact.

As for HDL and LDL: they are not types of cholesterol, which is a sort of alcohol, but are *lipoproteins*—packages that carry fats, cholesterol, and proteins to and from the liver to various organs. HDL (high density lipoprotein) and

LDL (low density lipoprotein) are supposedly the "good" and "bad" cholesterol, respectively. The term *density* refers to the proportion of protein in the packages. The less protein, the more fats and cholesterol (low density lipoprotein); the more protein, the less fats and cholesterol (high density lipoprotein). Think of HDL and LDL as little submarines. LDL is the little submarine that carries cholesterol, fats, and protein to the cells that need it. Sometimes a cell will have too much cholesterol. To handle this problem, the HDL submarine shows up and picks up the unwanted cholesterol as well any other excessive materials and takes it to the liver. That's why LDL (the cholesterol delivery submarine) is considered "bad," and the HDL (the cholesterol collection submarine) is considered "good." Both, of course, are just doing their jobs.

Because the National Cholesterol Education Committee has set the "desirable" level of total cholesterol to less than 200, high cholesterol can be diagnosed as a "disease" in half the population, which is probably why cholesterol-lowering drugs are among the top sellers in the U.S. (Most members of the Committee, by the way, have financial ties to the cholesterol-lowering drug manufacturers.)

The threshold for what is considered high cholesterol has been progressively lowered, each time without scientific evidence to support the lowering of the threshold. Of course, each time the threshold is lowered, millions more people become eligible for cholesterol-lowering medications—massively increasing the market size for the drugs and increasing the profits for pharmaceutical companies. (Henry Gadsen, a former chief executive of Merck, told *Fortune* magazine that it had long been his dream to make drugs for healthy people so that Merck would be able to "sell to everyone." This, of course, turns healthy people into patients.)

The most prescribed cholesterol-lowering drugs are called *statins*, which work by interrupting the chain of events by which our livers produce cholesterol. Because of this interruption, other substances, such as co-enzyme CoQ10 are also thwarted. CoQ10 is a cellular nutrient critical for maintaining the integrity of membranes for nerve conduction and muscle function. Depletion of CoQ10 and other substances that make up the chain cause a variety of side effects, the most common of which is muscle weakness and cramps. Many people who take statins also report problems with memory, depression and irritability, headaches, joint and abdominal pain, and tingling and numbness of extremities. The most serious and potentially fatal effect is rhabdomyolysis, in which muscle fibers break down and release their contents into the bloodstream. (Incidentally, a rare condition called familial hypercholesterolemia, may be a case where cholesterol-lowering drugs may be helpful. This genetic disease causes significantly elevated LDL.)

I get particularly upset when statin drugs are prescribed to old ladies, for whom the drugs have never proven beneficial (in fact, high cholesterol is protective in older women). I know of two older women on Lipitor who have fallen and broken bones. Another, the mother of a friend, lost her ability to walk. She died not long after. Martha

Weinman Lear, in her memoir of her heart attack, reports, "...I had been started on a high-cholesterol pill, which had caused me, and apparently millions of other users, to have severe leg cramps, and which had not, as was now clear, kept me from the absurdity of my new condition." These women should never have been prescribed the drugs, particularly since the drugs have not been shown to benefit anyone over 65 or women of any age, as revealed by an analysis of evidence from drug trials. Moreover, the incidence of falls among older people has steadily increased. The number of people over 65 who were treated in emergency departments for injuries from falls has increased 50 percent over a decade—perhaps because of the wide use of cholesterol-lowering drugs. If that weren't reason enough to avoid cholesterol-lowering drugs, research reported in the *British Medical Journal* (BMJ) has shown that people over 60 with the highest levels of LDL lived the longest.

Because of the nasty side effects of statins, pharmaceutical companies look for alternative drugs. Two of these, Praluent and Repatha, avoid the side effects. Trials for these drugs lowered LDL cholesterol and various types of heart attacks by 1.5 percent. But they did not decrease mortality. Plus, they cost $14,000 a year and must be taken for a lifetime. Another cholesterol-lowering drug (Evacetrapib) was found, in a phase two clinical trial, to increase HDL ("good") cholesterol levels by as much as 130% from baseline and reduce LDL ("bad") cholesterol levels by nearly 35%. However, the trial was "terminated early" because it "did not result in a lower rate of cardiovascular events than a placebo among patients," as reported in the *New England Journal of Medicine*. In other words, dramatically changing cholesterol levels had no effect on heart disease.

Studies of the relationship between cholesterol and heart disease are exhaustive and exhausting! I have read many books and articles on the subject and have come down on the side of The International Network of Cholesterol Skeptics (THINCS), a steadily growing group of scientists, physicians, academicians and science writers from various countries. As their website says, "Members of this group represent different views about the causation of atherosclerosis and cardiovascular disease, some of them are in conflict with others, but this is a normal part of science. *What we all oppose is that animal fat and high cholesterol play a role.* [My italics.]" In considering whether to recount for you the convincing results of their numerous studies, I decided that to do the topic justice would take reams of paper and bore you to tears.

Because it's been more than 20 years since my cholesterol has been measured, I have no idea what my readings are now. I don't worry about it.

5. Saturated Fat

Butter is considered saturated fat. We go through lots of butter at our house. My favorite clam chowder recipe calls for a stick and a half of it. I never buy non-fat or low-fat anything—always full fat. I don't worry about eating saturated fat.

The term "saturated" refers to fats—such as butter and animal fats—that are firm when refrigerated. Unfortunately, the word seems to imply that saturated fat is somehow "fattier" than other types of fat. But saturated simply describes the composition of the fat molecule: each carbon atom in the molecule is linked to two hydrogen atoms such that the carbon is "saturated" with hydrogen atoms. Yep, it's saturated with hydrogen. What's more, butter, like all fats, is a mixture of saturated, monounsaturated, and polyunsaturated fatty acids. For example, the fat component of a porterhouse steak is 51 percent monounsaturated (like olive oil), with only 45 percent saturated. The remaining four percent is polyunsaturated, like corn oil. Likewise, lard is only 40 percent saturated fat. Olive oil is 13.7 percent saturated fat, which is why it turns cloudy when refrigerated. A fat composed of all saturated molecules would be hard like candle wax. There's no such thing.

In the recent past, saturated fats and trans fats were lumped together in the various databases that researchers use to correlate dietary habits with disease. Big mistake: man-made trans fats are indeed bad for you and are implicated in a number of diseases. But because researchers didn't make the distinction between saturated and trans fats, they were able to find a correlation between disease and saturated fat consumption, giving saturated fats a bad name. While we now know better, the bad reputation lingers. Trans fats, by the way, are oils to which hydrogen has been added in a process called hydrogenation, giving it the same physical properties as animal-based fats, such as butter and lard. Researchers learned, after much damage had been done, that trans fats compromise many bodily functions, including hormone synthesis, immune function, insulin metabolism and tissue repair. They also significantly raise the risk of contracting heart disease.

Saturated fats do not clog arteries. They are either burned for fuel or stored in your fat cells. Your cells need saturated fat to help your body perform important chemical processes and make use of vitamins and minerals. For example, your body needs saturated fat to fully convert alpha-linolenic acid (one of the essential fatty acids) into the chemicals that control body temperature, stimulate smooth muscles, and other important control functions. Similarly, in order for calcium to be effectively incorporated into your bones, at least 50 percent of the fat you eat should be saturated. The fat in butter is a valuable source of A, D, K and E. These are fat-soluble vitamins that are essential for healthy bones and the proper development of your brain and nervous system.

The notion that saturated fat is bad for you is a myth that was debunked long ago by reputable scientists. For example, cardiologists L.A. Corr and M.F. Oliver, of the National Heart and Lung Institute, London, came to the following conclusions after reviewing results of a vast number of studies: "The commonly-held belief that the best diet for the prevention of coronary heart disease is one that is low in saturated fat and cholesterol is not supported by the available evidence from clinical trials...such diets do not reduce the risk of myocardial infarction or coronary or all-cause mortality." Many other studies come to the same conclusions. For example, reports in the *British Medical Journal* state that the data "do not support the strong association between intake of saturated fat and risk of coronary heart disease," and "do not support associations between intake of total fat, cholesterol, or specific types of fat and risk of stroke in men." Dr. Sylvan Lee Weinberg, past president of the American College of Cardiology writes, "Defense of the LF-HC [low-fat, high-carbohydrate] diet...is no longer tenable."

One researcher, Dr. Ivan Frantz Jr. of the University of Minnesota Medical School was determined to prove that replacing saturated fat, such as butter and other animal fats, with corn oil would protect people from heart disease and lower their mortality. From 1968 until 1973 he conducted a controlled clinical trial comparing diets containing saturated fats with those containing vegetable oils and no saturated fats. He enrolled 9,423 participants, ages 20 to 97, in his study. Because these participants lived in mental hospitals and a nursing home, their diets were strictly regulated. Half the subjects were fed meals rich in saturated fats from milk, cheese, and beef; the others ate a diet in which the fat consisted of corn oil. The result: those who ate the diet low in saturated fat reduced their cholesterol by an average of 14 percent, but the diet *did not reduce mortality*. In fact, the study showed that *the greater drop in cholesterol, the higher risk of death during the trial.* Even though this research was one of the largest controlled clinical trials ever conducted, the disappointed Dr. Frantz did not publish the results. Instead, he stored the data in his attic where it lay hidden away until after his death in 2009, at which time his son opened the dusty box and discovered the trove. As Dr. Frantz's son remarked, "My father definitely believed in reducing saturated fats," noting that his father was probably startled by what seemed to be no benefit in replacing saturated fat with vegetable oil.

While some nutritionists protest these findings, which were finally published in the *BMJ*, plenty of other scientists support them. For example, one scientist analyzed four similar trials in which vegetable oils were substituted for animal fats. Those trials also failed to show any reduction in mortality from heart disease. In 2013, Dr. Christopher Ramsden, who is a medical investigator for the National Institutes of Health, discovered a similar trial that had been carried out in Australia in the 1960s, but also had not been fully analyzed or published. Like the others, the results showed that those who replaced saturated fat with vegetable oils lowered their cholesterol but were also more likely to die from a heart attack than the control group who ate more saturated fat. "One would expect that the more you lowered cholesterol, the better the outcome. But in this case the opposite association was found. The greater degree of cholesterol-lowering was associated with a higher, rather than lower, risk of death."

The National Institutes of Health spent several hundred million dollars trying to demonstrate a connection between eating fat and getting heart disease, but never did find the connection. Dr. George Mann, former Director of the Framingham Heart Program called the belief that heart disease is caused by eating saturated fats and cholesterol "the greatest biomedical error of the twentieth century." Even though the connection has been proven untrue, the myth refuses to go away. In fact, the latest U.S. Dietary Guidelines for Americans continues to confirm its recommendation to limit saturated fats to 10 percent or less of total energy intake, ignoring scientific evidence from the last ten years that demonstrates a lack of rigorous evidence to support such recommendations.

Seeing saturated fats demonized in print is tiresome and annoying—not to mention wrong. What also annoys me is that labels on food products show the amount of saturated fat but not the amounts of monounsaturated or polyunsaturated fats, implying that you must be on the lookout for saturated fats.

While I was writing this chapter, *The American Journal of Clinical Nutrition* published one of the largest and most rigorous trials of low carbohydrate/high fat diets to date. In commenting about the new study, Dr. Dariush Mozaffarian, a cardiologist and dean of the Friedman School of Nutrition Science and Policy at Tufts University, said "It's a well-controlled trial that shows that eating lower carb and more saturated fat is actually good for you...Most Americans still believe that low-fat foods are healthier for them, and this trial shows that at least for these outcomes, the high-fat, low-carb group did better." The test subjects who ate the most saturated fat (21 percent of their daily calories) got the best scores on the biomarkers that indicate resistance to heart attacks, strokes, diabetes, and inflammation.

Similarly, a previous large study published in *The Lancet*, found that eating two or more servings of whole fat dairy foods, such as milk, yogurt and cheese, reduced the risk of heart disease. The study included 136,384 people in 21 countries who were followed for an average of nine years. The results showed a 22 percent lower risk of heart disease, a 34 percent lower risk of stroke, and a 23 percent lower risk of death from cardiovascular disease.

After analyzing studies that focus on the "diet heart hypothesis," researchers J. Bruce German and Cora J. Dillard state, in the *American Journal of Clinical Nutrition* (September 2004), "after 50 years of research, there was no evidence that a diet low in saturated fat prolongs life." Moreover, these authors note that, "if saturated fatty acids were of no value or were harmful to humans, evolution would probably not have established within the mammary gland the means to produce saturated fatty acids—butyric, caproic, caprylic, capric, lauric, myristic, palmitic, and stearic acids—that provide a source of nourishment to ensure the growth, development, and survival of mammalian offspring."

Like me, Mother Nature approves of eating saturated fat.

6. Medications

For years, before setting out for golf, I took a couple of Advil (I play golf twice a week). I'd occasionally take it on other days as needed for the aches and pains of my 85-year-old body. It did help. After years of this regimen, I started having occasional bouts of acid reflux and heartburn, which, I later discovered, can be caused by Advil. I quit taking Advil and the acid reflux and heartburn stopped. The other problem with Advil and other non-steroidal anti-inflammatories, such as Aleve, Celebrex, and aspirin, is that they suppress our immune systems. Inflammation occurs when your immune system sends out cells to fight bacteria or heal an injury. You need your immune system to work, so it's best not to overdo.

As with Advil, the thing that makes me wary of taking drugs is their side effects, which can range from annoying to life-threatening. My husband quit taking statins (cholesterol-lowering drugs) because of terrible muscle cramps. Statins work by inhibiting an enzyme that's required for producing cholesterol. But the inhibition of this enzyme blocks the synthesis of co-enzyme Q-10, a critical cellular nutrient that, when deficient, causes muscle weakness and cramps.

My sister, who is two years older than I, took a blood pressure medicine called hydrochlorothiazide, a diuretic (a drug that makes you pee). After taking it a while, she developed pain in her feet, a symptom of gout. (Your body naturally produces uric acid, which normally dissolves in your blood and passes through your kidneys into your urine. Because diuretics increase urination and reduce the amount of fluid in your body, the acid can build up and form needle-like crystals that cause gout.) She quit taking the drug and the gout-like symptoms disappeared.

As you might imagine, there's also the fact that different people respond differently to the same medication. I read a case study about a woman who was being treated for ulcerative colitis with a prescription of sulfasalazine (a combination of a sulfa drug and aspirin). She got desperately ill, so she went to the hospital and was put into intensive care, where doctors discovered that she had bone marrow suppression, meaning a decrease in production of red and white blood cells. They were pretty sure she had leukemia, but it turned out she was allergic to sulfasalazine.

Prescription drugs, even when properly prescribed, rank fourth along with stroke as a leading cause of death: about 128,000 people die every year from drugs prescribed for them. In addition, prescription drugs cause about 1.9 million hospitalizations a year, and about 81 million adverse reactions. For people over 65, 12 percent of hospitalizations are linked to medications. An FDA study

46

states that "adverse drug reactions are one of the leading causes of morbidity and mortality in health care." The reason for the high mortality rate is the high prescription rate for patients looking for relief. In 2016, over four billion prescriptions were filled in the US. That's about 12 prescriptions for every person in the country. Sixty-four percent of all patient visits to physicians result in prescriptions (this was in 2000). Adverse drug reactions increase exponentially after a patient is on four or more medications.

You may be old enough to remember thalidomide. In the 1950s and early 1960s the drug was given to pregnant women as a cure for nausea. Unfortunately, it caused severe birth defects in their children, most notably truncated or missing limbs. Because of the dire consequences of this drug, in 1962 the government enacted the Kefauver-Harris amendment to the Federal Food, Drug and Cosmetic Act. The new amendment requires drug makers to satisfy the FDA that their products are safe and effective before they go on sale. (I was astounded to learn that, before 1962, drugs could be sold without any data to support their claims of safety and efficacy.) When the law went into effect, more than 100,000 drugs already on the market needed to be reviewed. To streamline the process, if a drug's components had been deemed to be safe and effective, it could be used under specific conditions without further review. But about a third of the drugs have still not undergone a final review process. That is, hundreds of over-the-counter drugs have not yet been determined to be safe and effective.

Just because a drug has been approved by the FDA doesn't mean it's safe. Even after the FDA approves a drug, the risk of serious adverse reactions is one in three. The most infamous example was Vioxx, an FDA-approved drug that experts say caused about 120,000 traumatic cardiovascular events and 40,000 deaths. The drug is no longer on the market. It turns out that new prescription drugs have a one in five chance of causing serious reactions after they have been approved. For this reason, experienced physicians recommend not taking new drugs unless they have been on the market for at least five years. It takes that long to determine whether they are safe.

To gain FDA approval for a new drug, pharmaceutical companies must show that it outperforms placebos in two independent studies. This is not easy. For example, more than 90 percent of pain medications fail in the final stage of drug trials. In other words, most drugs did not perform better than placebos. Every clinical trial is actually a study of the placebo effect. (Placebo is Latin for 'I will please' and refers to a treatment that appears real but has no therapeutic benefit. For example, in clinical trials, one group of test subjects may be given a sugar pill instead of the medication being tested.)

The placebo effect is powerful. It can evoke a real neurobiological healing response, using the pathways that affect bodily sensations, symptoms, and emotions. As one scientist remarked, "It seems that if the mind can be persuaded, the body can sometimes act accordingly." Healing rituals and acts of caring can also affect the healing response. The brain translates the act of caring into

48

physical healing, turning on the biological processes that relieve pain, reduce inflammation, and promote health.

Scientists have recently discovered that responses to placebos vary among people depending on their genetic makeup. A particular snippet of our genome governs the production of an enzyme, called COMT, that affects people's response to pain and painkillers. Some people have weak placebo responses and some have strong responses. For years, scientists thought that the placebo effect was the work of the imagination. Now, with the use of imaging machines, they can see the brain lighting up when some test subjects are given a sugar pill. Those people who are strong placebo responders show consistent patterns of brain activation. If drug companies can weed out the strong placebo responders from their trials, the drugs being tested are less likely to be shown as being no better than a placebo.

Most of the new drugs offer few advantages over old ones. Independent reviews by expert teams in France, Canada, and the Netherlands have concluded that of the 946 new products released between 2002 and 2010, only two were breakthroughs and only 13 represented a real therapeutic advance. The remaining 85 to 89 percent of the new drugs offered little or no clinical advantage. And yet these new drugs continue to flood the market. The reason that new drugs offer few advantages over old ones is that companies just tinker a bit with their existing drugs, then begin pushing these "new drugs." (I read about one man who pried the coating off a "new" drug to find the old drug underneath. The "improvement" was merely the coating.)

Nevertheless, pharmaceutical sales and profits are soaring, largely as a result of raising prices and getting more physicians to prescribe more and newer drugs. Naturally, the new drugs are far more costly than the drugs they replace.

The wrongdoing of big pharma is so vast that many books have been written about the ways in which drug companies deceive us. One good one is *The Truth About the Drug Companies: How They Deceive Us and What To Do About It.* The author is Marcia Angell, M.D., who is the former editor in chief of *The New England Journal of Medicine.* She describes the pharmaceutical industry as having "moved very far from its original high purpose of discovering and producing useful new drugs" to becoming "a marketing machine to sell drugs of dubious benefit." The companies now "use their wealth and power to co-opt every institution that might stand in its way, including the U.S. Congress, the Food and Drug Administration, academic medical centers and the medical profession itself." Since the early 1980s—with few exceptions--pharmaceutical companies have consistently ranked as the most profitable companies in the United States (more than $200 billion a year). Their high profits deserve scrutiny.

Here are some of the ways big pharma deceives:

- **Over charging**. The cost of the drug is unrelated to the costs of research and development, as they would have us believe. Instead, the costs, which are continually rising, are based on what the public is willing to pay.

- **Manipulating research findings to make drugs look good.** As much as 90 percent of published medical information—the kind of information that doctors rely on—is flawed, according to the world's foremost expert on the credibility of medical research.
- **Rewarding doctors to promote their drugs**. Companies spend more than four billion dollars nationwide in payments to doctors as incentives for attending industry-sponsored conferences, as well as for promoting their drugs at the conferences.
- **Rewarding doctors to prescribe their drugs**. The rewards to doctors range from meals to generous honoraria for speaking at conferences. As a rule, the doctors who prescribe the most are rewarded the most.
- **Promoting old drugs as new**. Most of the new drugs approved by the FDA are "me too" drugs— old drugs whose molecules have been only slightly altered so they can appear as new. They are more expensive but no more effective than the old models.
- **Passing off their professionally written articles as the work of academics**. Drug companies pay professional writers to produce academic papers according to the companies' specifications, then reward the academics for adding their names to them.

- **Passing off marketing as "education**." The so-called "education" programs come out of drug companies' marketing budgets, which, collectively, in 2001, amounted to $19 billion. By masquerading marketing as education, big pharma can evade legal constraints on marketing activities.

The British Medical Association awarded Dr. Peter C Gøtzsche first prize in the "basis of health care" category for his book, *Deadly Medicines and Organised Crime. How Big Pharma Has Corrupted Healthcare*. Among other things, Gøtzsche enumerates the corrupt practices of pharmaceutical companies (years 2003-2013). These are big names, such as Eli-Lilly and Pfizer, both of which were charged with fraudulent marketing. Johnson & Johnson was also charged with illegal marketing. Eleven additional companies were listed with similar charges of wrongdoing, including bribery, kickbacks, and lies. To corroborate, an organization called Access to Medicine Index found that "18 out of 20 companies were the subject of settlements or fines for corrupt behavior, unethical marketing or breaches of competition law. Collectively, companies were found to have been accountable for almost 100 separate breaches...The majority of these (89%) concerned improper marketing, bribery and corruption." Incidentally, even though some business practices of Pfizer and Johnson & Johnson have been questionable, I trust their Covid vaccines.

When a drug's U.S. patent expires, usually after about 20 years, the drug's price drops. Moreover, manufacturers other than the initial developer may take advantage of an abbreviated approval process to introduce lower-priced generic versions. In most uses, generics are clinically equivalent to the original branded drug. But many of the generic drug manufacturers are not trustworthy. For example, in 2007 scores of kidney patients across the United States died from allergic reactions to the blood thinner heparin. The generic heparin, which was manufactured in China, was contaminated.

In the U.S., imports from India make up 40 percent of all the generics we use; 80 percent of the active ingredients in both generic and brand-name medications come from India and China. In other words, the Asian companies have merged with Big Pharma. I suppose this wouldn't be so bad if the drugs were always pure. But they're not. The FDA is supposed to regulate the industry by inspecting production practices and testing facilities and by exhaustively checking records. But inspection visits are rare and, until recently, the manufacturers are given plenty of notice before inspectors arrive, giving corporate officers time to destroy failed quality test results and fabricate documents that show successful tests. Some plants have even built fake production and testing areas that are kept pristine just for inspection purposes. I've learned that FDA inspectors themselves avoid taking drugs made overseas. As a Ghanaian creator of a drug verification program noted, "All medicines are poisonous. It's only under the most controlled conditions that they do good."

I know this all sounds very alarming. Sorry. Now I've made you worry. Surely some drugs are helpful—even lifesaving. But for me, I'll just trust my body to take care of itself.

7. Food

As a rule, I don't pay much attention to nutrition studies as reported in the press. Nutritional research is plagued with credibility problems. This is partly because the world of scientific research is competitive. Post-doctoral candidates compete for fewer jobs. Grant money and livelihoods depend on getting research published. Journals select articles that make splashy news, and the popular press publishes the most newsworthy studies. For this reason, many researchers go for attention-grabbing results. This was the case for a respected and often-quoted founder of the Food and Brand Lab at Cornell University. In 2019, he was booted from his position because of "academic misconduct in his research and scholarship, including misreporting of research data." His studies have been cited more than 20,000 times. Fifteen of those studies have been retracted. He's not alone in his misconduct, just a big name who was busted.

What this has led to, in the words of one researcher, is an "epidemic of fraud." The "fraud" in this case consists of such deceptions as leaving out contradictory data, cutting corners, or even making up data. One deceptive practice is "data dredging" whereby researchers run exhaustive analyses on data sets then cherry pick the "findings" that produce exciting results. Another problem is weak experiment protocols in which the researcher incorrectly assumes cause and effect; that is, he or she concludes that A causes B, when in fact some other factor may be causing B.

Dr. Ancel Keys, an influential scientist whose popular book, *How to Eat Well and Stay Well the Mediterranean Way*, provides another example of fraudulent science. In the 1950s he undertook some studies that supposedly implicated saturated fat and cholesterol in heart disease. But his study methods were deeply flawed. For example, he collected data from twenty-countries but, because only data from seven of the countries supported his hypothesis, he tossed out the contradictory data. Similarly, he used the dietary data of less than five percent of the total sample— the data that supported his hypothesis. Even though subsequent large-scale clinical trial data from around the world refuted Keys' findings, his influence persists. In 1992, the U.S. government's nutritional guidelines indicated that the bulk of your diet should consist of carbohydrates "bread, rice, cereal, pasta, 6-11 servings." (It has since been modified.) Keys himself, at age ninety-four, acknowledged that dietary cholesterol is unrelated to heart disease. Too late. For years, millions of people stopped eating eggs because of their high cholesterol content.

The Mediterranean diet continues to be popular. It promotes grains, vegetables, fruits, legumes, nuts, beans, fish, and unsaturated fats such as olive oil, and a low intake of meat and dairy foods. In an exhaustive study involving almost a million people, researchers found that "the totality of evidence did not favor the Mediterranean diet for cardiovascular outcomes." There's nothing wrong with it; it's neither favorable nor harmful—just "...a neutral diet from a cardiovascular perspective," according to Dr. Safi U. Khan, lead author of the study. The same study, which included rigorous randomized trials, found that eating less fat, including saturated fat, had no impact on cardiovascular health or mortality.

I must admit that I do pay attention to studies that support my biases. Case in point: in 2018, a study published in *The Lancet* showed that eating two or more servings of full fat dairy was "associated with lower rates of cardiovascular disease and mortality." The study was huge (136,384 people) and went on for nine years. It was controlled for age, sex, smoking, physical activity, and other factors. The journal report went so far as to state that "some saturated fats may be beneficial to cardiovascular health, and dairy products may also contain other potentially beneficial compounds." Because the results of this study go against conventional wisdom, it didn't make headlines. I was lucky enough to find a brief mention of it in *The New York Times*. I like that one.

Here's another one I liked: whole grain bread is no better for you than white bread. I trust this myth-breaking idea because it comes from Nathan Myhrvold, former

Chief Technology Officer for Microsoft. He holds a doctorate in theoretical and mathematical physics from Princeton University, did postdoctoral work with Stephen Hawking, and also acquired a culinary diploma from École de Cuisine La Varenne, in France. After leaving Microsoft, he became interested in food science and has spent many years enmeshed in the study of food, which includes establishing an elaborate test kitchen. One of his studies compared whole grain bread and white bread. He found no evidence that whole grain bread is better for you than white bread and, in fact, found some "evidence to the contrary." After sifting through fifty years of studies, his team found that all types of breads have pretty much the same result in your body. The theory has always been that the bran is the healthy part of the bread because it contains more fiber and vitamins. (In processing flour, the bran is separated from the inner wheat kernel. With white bread, the bran is left out; with whole wheat bread, the bran is put back into the flour.) Myhrvold says that when studied on a nutrient-by-nutrient basis, whole wheat bread might be slightly better because the bran contains manganese, phosphorus, and selenium, but that these components are "generally not important in the sense that they're not things that most people run a deficit of." Moreover, our bodies don't absorb many of the vitamins and minerals in raw grain. Even worse, a compound in bran called phytates can bind to some of the potentially beneficially minerals to block their absorption—it's called the anti-nutrient effect. The other supposed benefit of bran is that it causes the starch to break down more slowly, preventing sugar spike and delivering a longer, steadier flow of glucose into the body. Myhrvold's response: because whole grain bread is only 11 percent bran, the effect on blood glucose is minimal. So now I don't have to feel guilty about eating white ciabatta bread, my favorite.

As to the gluten in bread, you don't need to worry about that either, unless you have celiac disease. People with celiac disease have an immune reaction triggered by eating gluten. Symptoms include diarrhea, abdominal pain, weight loss, bloating, and an itchy rash. Gluten is a protein found in many grains, such as wheat, barley, and rye. As the Senior Faculty Editor of *Harvard Health Publishing* tells us, "There is no compelling evidence that a gluten-free diet will improve health or prevent disease." In fact, he adds, "Gluten-free foods are commonly less fortified with folic acid, iron and other nutrients than regular, gluten-containing foods." I pay no attention to whether a food item contains gluten.

I also don't worry about the "sell by" dates printed on food packages. I just don't care about such things. My one exception is fresh bean sprouts. They only last a couple of days, so I check packages to find the furthest-out date. I know that other people do examine those sell-by labels, so I decided to find out who was right: me or other people. Turns out it's me.

In 2013, the Harvard Food Law and Policy Clinic and the Natural Resources Defense Council produced an exhaustive, sixty-one-page report called "The Dating Game: How Confusing Food Date Labels Lead to Food

Waste in America." Here's what I learned (quoted phrases come from the report):

"Sell by:" "There is no direct correlation between food safety and date labels." As a rule, it merely "provides information to retailers for stock control…The use of these dates does not advance public health in a meaningful way." In other words, the labels have nothing to do with food safety.

"Use by" or "best if used by:" Typically, these labels are an "estimate of a date after which food will no longer be at its highest quality." Manufacturers and retailers are "free to define shelf-life according to their own market standards…The fact that consumers and stores throw away products unnecessarily can lead to increased profits for manufacturers if consumers are purchasing more products and doing so more often…some manufacturers may artificially shorten stated shelf lives for marketing reasons." In other words, the more you throw away, the more replacements you need to buy.

Regulations: The federal government has no regulations that control date labels. Some states regulate the labels, others don't. For example, New York does not require date labels to be put on any food products, but neighbor New Jersey does. Furthermore, there's no legal definition for the "sell by" and "use by" terms.

"Sell by" and "use by" labels may be a leading reason why Americans throw out tons of perfectly good food each year. In the U.S., we toss out about 40 percent of the food we produce, which amounts to a $165 billion in wasted food each year. For a family, this waste costs the average American family of four $2,275 a year.

We don't waste much food at our house. Of course, I throw away food that's truly bad, but I trust my senses to determine if food is edible. That is, I taste and sniff. I used this method after we had to evacuate our home in the Santa Cruz Mountains for two-and-a-half weeks because of the 2020 CZU Lightning Complex fire. Even though we took a lot of the food from our refrigerator to our evacuation place, we still had to leave plenty behind. During the period we were gone, our home had no electricity and thus no refrigeration. When we returned, our refrigerator was a horror, mostly because we'd left some meat behind. After throwing out the truly horrific stuff and thoroughly cleaning the refrigerator, I started going through the food that wasn't obviously spoiled. I discovered that much of it was fine. Most people just threw everything away. In fact, our town installed a dumpster to handle all of this thrown-out food. A lot of people even threw out their refrigerators.

In tasting and sniffing the contents of our refrigerator, the most surprising finding was the almost-full quart of pomegranate juice. I tasted it. It was fine! I started examining and tasting other items, such as olives. They were also fine. I ended up keeping most of the jars that sit in the refrigerator door—such items as pickles, capers, mustards, hot sauces, and everything else that was either salty, vinegary, or spicy hot. I guess that's sort of a no-brainer, when you think about it.

I've never refrigerated items such as tomatoes, onions, potatoes, and fruit. But I did a little research and discovered that in addition to the salty, vinegary, and spicy items I've mentioned, you don't need to refrigerate eggs (unless cracked, of course). You don't need to refrigerate syrups because spoilage bacteria can't grow when the sugar content is high. You also don't need to refrigerate butter—which I knew. I always leave one stick on the kitchen counter but refrigerate the rest, which I'll keep doing just for convenience. On an earlier occasion, I also learned, thanks to friends who had been house-sitting, that you don't need to refrigerate peanut butter. It's so much easier to spread at room temperature! Even though they don't require refrigeration, all my mustards, sauces, pickles, and such are still in the door of the refrigerator. I'm used to them being there and know where to find them.

Speaking of expiration dates, I was cleaning out the medicine cabinet the other day and came across some prednisone that a friend had given me over 20 years ago. Prednisone is a powerful corticosteroid anti-inflammatory drug that I've taken to combat poison ivy. In that case, it was miraculous. Anyhow, I took one just to see what would happen. The answer: nothing. Dang. I had a newly pulled muscle plus other aches and pains to test it on. I guess 20 years is pushing it. Maybe not. Some scientists at the California Poison Control System tested the effectiveness of eight drugs that had been sitting around unopened in pharmacies a full *28 to 40 years past their expiration dates.* They used a mass spectrometer to analyze how much of the active ingredients remained in the pills. Of the 14 active ingredients, 12 were still at a high enough concentration to qualify as "acceptable potency." Some of these ingredients included acetaminophen, codeine, hydrocodone, methaqualone (Quaaludes!), and caffeine. Aspirin as an active ingredient didn't make the cut.

At any rate, many drugs are just fine after their expiration date. The expiration date on a drug is usually one to five years after it was manufactured. But those dates are often set *arbitrarily*. The FDA doesn't require pharmaceutical makers to test how long the active ingredients will last. So basically, they don't really know.

The poison control researchers are all for extending expiration dates for many drugs. In fact, the Shelf Life Extension Program (SLEP) does just that for drugs in federal stockpiles. The program, which is administered by the U.S. Department of Defense in cooperation with the FDA, acknowledges that the actual shelf life of drugs may be longer than their stated expiration date. They allow drugs in federal stockpiles to be retained for up to 278 months if tests show they are still potent. Some of the ingredients remained good for 480 months—so far.

But I digress. In addition to not worrying about "sell by" dates, I don't care whether the food I eat has been genetically modified. GMO (GMO—genetically modified organism) plants have had their genes altered using DNA from different species of living organisms, bacteria, or viruses to get desired traits such as resistance to disease or tolerance of drought and pesticides. For example, in the 1990s, the ringspot virus decimated nearly half the papaya crops in Hawaii. Now, 77 percent of the crop has been genetically engineered to resist the virus. Most of our processed foods contain GMOs, but most fruits and vegetables do not. Until just recently, no meat, fish, or poultry products approved for direct human consumption have been bioengineered, although most of the feed for livestock and fish is derived from genetically modified corn, alfalfa, and other biotech grains.

Though I have no problem with GMO food, plenty of people do. Even though the National Academy of Sciences has declared that GMOs are safe, the market for products certified to be non-GMO has increased more than 70-fold since 2010. Because of fear of the unknown, consumers are willing to pay 20 percent more to avoid GMO foods. Of course, through crossbreeding, almost everything we eat has had its DNA altered extensively. But it takes much longer to alter foodstuffs this way—150 years in some cases.

Seventeen European countries and nearly all countries in sub-Saharan Africa, which follow Europe's lead, have banned the cultivation of genetically modified crops. In some conspiracy-theory-prone African countries people believe that eating GMO foods will turn you into a homosexual! Not only do GMO plants not turn you into a homosexual, but the worldwide scientific consensus concludes that GMO foods are as safe to eat as conventionally cultivated food. More importantly, plants that have been genetically modified for, say, insect resistance, have caused a 40 percent reduction in insecticide use worldwide. Ditto for fungicides. However, because of the bans, farmers in Tanzania, for example, have had their cassava crops wiped out by brown-streak disease, while farmers in neighboring Uganda are growing cassava with complete resistance to the virus. As Mark Lynas, political director of the Cornell Alliance for Science says, "Thanks to Europe's Coalition of the Ignorant, we are witnessing a historic injustice perpetrated by the well fed on the food insecure."

Unfortunately, the creation of GMO food was started in a rather unsavory way. Monsanto introduced the first GMO in 1996—an herbicide-resistant soybean. Farmers could slather their soybean fields with Monsanto's herbicide Roundup without harming their Monsanto-engineered soybean crop. Monsanto became the largest producer of genetically engineered seeds, including corn, sugar beets, and canola. (By the way, farmers are not allowed to save seeds from these crops. At one time, Monsanto had a 75-person team dedicated to investigating seed-saving farmers, who could then be prosecuted on charges of intellectual-property infringement.) Unfortunately, this sleazy beginning tarnished the whole GMO technology, which has the potential to improve food production where it's most needed. For example, Golden Rice was created by a pair of university researchers hoping to combat vitamin A deficiency, a devastating ailment that causes blindness in millions of people in Africa and Asia annually.

You may be one of those people who have a legitimate worry about certain foods. I have a friend who passes out if she eats strawberries; another who becomes ill by eating garlic; another who is allergic to artichokes. Many people cannot eat certain types of shellfish. Because of differences in genetic makeup, people react differently to different foods. In the same way, medicines affect people differently. For example, certain cancer medicines help some people but not others. Add to that your gut bacteria, which vary a great deal among people, and which affect not only your physical health but also your mental health. Unfortunately, researchers haven't nailed down ways to determine what foods or medicines are either beneficial or toxic to you specifically. For now, you're stuck with trial and error.

Speaking of which, you may have discovered that certain foods don't "sit well" with you. Apparently, there's a group of carbohydrates that are not well absorbed in the small intestine and may cause you intestinal problems. In addition to being poorly absorbed during the digestive process, these foods are rapidly fermented by bacteria that live in your gut and can pull fluid into the gut. The fluid load plus the gas produced by the bacteria are what usually cause the discomfort. These problematic foods fall under the heading of FODMAP, an acronym that stands for Fermentable Oligosaccharides Disaccharides Monosaccharides And Polyols. The list of foods is long (see the appendix).

Scientists are continually learning about the ways in which our gut bacteria (microbiome) affect our health. Now they are trying to individualize this information by pinpointing the health effects of particular foods eaten by particular people, assuming bacteria are accomplices. Case in point: cardiologist Dr. Eric Topol participated in a two-week experiment to determine which foods created spikes in his blood-glucose levels (glycemic response). Such spikes are thought to be indicators of diabetes risk. In the experiment, a smartphone app tracked every morsel of food he ate, every beverage he drank, and every medication he took. He submitted a stool sample to get a reading of his gut microbiome and wore a sensor that monitored his blood-glucose level. This information was analyzed to determine which foods, and the bacteria's actions on those foods, created spikes. (By the way, a substantial portion of healthy people have high glucose levels after eating.) Dr. Topol was surprised at the outcome of his test. He got an A for cheesecake, but C- in whole-wheat fig bars; an A+ for strawberries but a C in grapefruit; an A+ for mixed nuts, but C for veggie burgers; A+ for bratwurst, but C- for oatmeal. In other words, cheesecake did not spike his glucose levels, but whole-wheat fig bars did—and so forth.

Blood glucose spikes are the first objective proof that people respond differently to eating the same food. In collecting billions of data points on thousands of people, researchers have found that more than a hundred factors are involved in glucose spikes. Surprisingly, they learned that *food was not the key determinant*. Instead, it was the *gut bacteria*. One of these studies, called Predict, followed over 1,100 mostly healthy adults in the United States and Britain, including hundreds of identical and nonidentical twins. As Dr. Topol's experience illustrated, different people can have wildly different metabolic responses to the same foods, mediated in part by the kinds of microbes residing in their guts. Dr. Andrew T. Chan, a co-author of the study and professor of medicine at Harvard Medical School, remarked, "What we found in our study was that the same diet in two different individuals does not lead to the same microbiome, and it does not lead to the same metabolic response. There is a lot of variation."

Obviously, the takeaway from such studies is that there is no such thing as a universal diet—one that is right for everyone. Our bodies, and especially our microbiomes, are simply too complex. For one thing, we harbor 40 trillion bacteria and 1,000 species in our guts—probably unique mixtures of these critters in every person. Dr. Topol, for example, has way more *Bacteriodes stercoris* than the general population. In comparison, my most abundant bacteria are in the Prevotella bacteria family. As to the right food for you: you'll probably never know, unless, of course, accurate tests become widely available.

Maybe what you need to be eating is dirt. Hundreds of thousands of people around the world eat dirt. Not just any dirt will do. In the U.S. southeastern states, such as Georgia, a white clay called kaolin is the dirt of choice. Apparently, it's mostly women who crave dirt, especially pregnant women. "Every time I get pregnant, I get a craving—I have to eat it," says one woman who has given birth to four healthy babies. Some medical professionals believe that minerals in certain clays are especially beneficial for pregnant women. As one said, "Mineral demand goes up substantially during pregnancy. Soil is nature's multi-mineral supply." Other researchers believe that eating dirt while pregnant strengthens both the mother's and child's immune systems. It can also have a calming effect on the mother's gastrointestinal system, since the clay (also found in Maalox and Rolaids) contains antacid compounds. Because clay absorbs toxins, people in traditional cultures cook food such as potatoes and acorns in clay as a way of protecting against the toxic alkaloids and tannic acids that would otherwise make these foods inedible. If you're hankering for some kaolin clay, you can buy it on the internet.

There's a clay deposit in Canada that has been found to contain powerful antibiotics. In fact, solutions of the clay can kill 16 different strains of multi-drug-resistant bacteria—such as *Staphylococcus aurea*—that commonly infect hospital patients. As one scientist noted, the antimicrobial clay provides "new hope in a battle that the medical community is currently not winning." Actually, the Canadian find is not new. Natives of the region, the Heiltsuk, have used the clay for medicinal purposes for generations.

One thing we should all be concerned about is eating enough fiber. I think most of us thought that the value of eating fiber-rich foods was for the roughage it provides—indigestible bulk that keeps food moving through your digestive tract. It turns out that eating fiber is way more important than that. It feeds billions of bacteria in our guts, keeping them happy and, in turn, keeping our intestines and immune systems in good working order.

Here's how it works: enzymes in our bodies break down food molecules, enabling us to digest the food. But our bodies make a limited range of enzymes, so we can't break down many of the tough compounds in plants. That's where the bacteria come in. Some of the bacteria have the enzymes needed to break down various kinds of fibers—the kind present in vegetables, fruits, and nuts. Scientists have found that diets low in the fiber result in a variety of negative effects. For one thing, certain populations of bacteria crash; many common species become rare and rare species become common. Without a steady stream of chemical signals from bacteria, the intestinal cells slow their production of mucus as well as bacteria-killing poisons that are needed to wipe out the bacteria that get too close to the gut wall—a condition that kicks the immune system into high gear. In the words of one of the scientists, "The gut is always precariously balanced between trying to contain these organisms and not to overreact. It could be a tipping point between health and disease." Dr. Rob Knight, the founder of the American Gut Project, has concluded that the more diverse our diets, plant-wise, the more diverse our gut microbiomes: "The single greatest predictor of a healthy gut microbiome is the diversity of plants in one's diet." Knight's recommendation is to eat *thirty different plants a week*—a number that he found was the greatest predictor of microbial diversity. According to Knight, this doesn't require being a vegetarian. I've tried counting the variety fruits and vegetables I eat. It turns out that reaching thirty isn't that hard.

8. Supplements

I don't take any of food supplements. Experts agree: the December 2013 issue of *Annals of Internal Medicine* published an editorial titled "Enough Is Enough: Stop Wasting Money on Vitamin and Mineral Supplements." The authors were from Johns Hopkins University and other august institutions. The researchers performed a thorough investigation of clinical trials that tested the usefulness of supplements. Their conclusion: "We believe that the case is closed— supplementing the diet of well-nourished adults with (most) mineral or vitamin supplements has no clear benefit and might even be harmful."

Before I became enlightened, I tried glucosamine-chondroitin in hopes that it would reduce my developing arthritis. I tried it for many months and noticed no difference. I have since learned that a randomized trial of more than 1,500 people showed no improvement through using this supplement.

At one time, I tried taking fish oil supplements, although I hated taking them because I tend to gag on large pills. I was happy to learn from reliable sources that fish oil supplements have no value for preventing heart disease. For example, according to the National Institutes of Health: "Omega-3s in supplement form have not been shown to protect against heart disease." Former president of the AMA, Robert Eckel has also stated that nearly all studies regarding fish oil supplements show no benefit at all. Dr. John Ioannidis, Professor of Medicine at Stanford University, specializes in uncovering flaws in published research. He long ago showed the worthlessness of fish oil supplements. He says, "These claims do not easily die away." Indeed, every year people in the U.S. spend $1.2 billion a year on fish oil and similar supplements. You are probably among them. I say this because the use of fish oil supplements has quadrupled over the last five years and because nearly one in five older adults now take them. "There's a major disconnect," says researcher Dr. Andrew Grey. "The sales are going up despite the progressive accumulation of trials that show no effect."

Furthermore, fish oil supplements are largely unregulated. Tests performed on 30 top-selling fish oil supplements found that six of those products contained 30 percent less omega-3 fatty acids than stated on their labels. Tests that looked for two particular omega-3's (DHA and EPA) found that, on average, these fats were 14 percent less than listed on the product packaging. Although fish oil supplements have not been shown to be harmful, they can

72

cause bleeding if you take blood thinners such as Coumadin, or even aspirin.

Vitamin D is another popular supplement. We need vitamin D because it increases our intestinal absorption of calcium, magnesium, and phosphorus and makes our bones strong. We get most of the vitamin through a synthesis that occurs on our skin. The synthesis is a complicated process involving a chemical that resides in our skin combined with exposure to the sun (ultraviolet light). (Vitamin D is found in only a few foods, such as egg yolks, oily fish and milk fortified with vitamin D.) Because many people have little exposure to sunlight, especially those living in northern areas in the winter, some investigators became concerned that large swaths of the population were not getting enough of the vitamin. It turns out this is not true.

In 2007, one influential doctor published a paper asserting that blood levels of vitamin D below 29 nanograms per milliliter of blood leads to an increased risk of cancer, autoimmune disease, diabetes, schizophrenia, depression, poor lung capacity and wheezing. (He's also published books.) Word got around. Soon "there was a vitamin D bandwagon," in the words of Mayo Clinic doctor. Doctors began incorporating vitamin D tests into the general evaluation of patients. Commercial labs immediately began describing levels of 20 to 30 nanograms as insufficient—and many continue to do so. The number of blood tests for vitamin D among Medicare beneficiaries increased 83-fold from 2000 to 2010. Among those with commercial insurance, testing rates rose 2.5-fold from 2009 to 2014.

In the meantime, a number of scientists performed multiple studies to verify the doctor's claim, which turned out not to be true. After conducting many trials with thousands of test subjects, scientists found that those who took vitamin D supplements were no better off than those who took placebos. After reviewing the studies, the Institute of Medicine prepared a report stating that there's no benefit for healthy people to have blood levels above 20 nanograms of vitamin D per milliliter of blood. After becoming convinced that the tests weren't necessary, one doctor tried to discourage her patients from being tested. "But," she said, "people were used to vitamin D monitoring, like with cholesterol. They wanted to know what their number is."

To finally put the vitamin D issue to rest, the federal government funded the first large randomized controlled study of the vitamin's effects. The report, which involved more than 25,000 participants, was published in July, 2022, in the *New England Journal of Medicine*. The study found that vitamin D pills taken with or without calcium have no effect on bone fracture rates, even for those with osteoporosis. In addition to finding that the supplements do not protect you from fractures, it also does not prevent falls, cancer or cardiovascular disease, nor does it improve cognitive functioning, reduce atrial fibrillation, reduce migraine frequency, improve stroke outcomes, protect against macular degeneration, or reduce knee pain. As the report states, "providers should stop screening for 25-hydroxyvitamin D levels and people should stop taking vitamin D supplements in order to prevent major diseases or extend life." There's no reason to be tested for vitamin D, even if you live in Maine. It's just another unnecessary test.

I don't use probiotic supplements either. The technical definition of probiotics is "live microorganisms that, when administered in adequate amounts, confer a health benefit to the host." Most scientific studies have not found any health benefits from consuming them, either in supplements or in foods such as yogurt and sauerkraut. Dr. Pieter Cohen, an assistant professor at Harvard Medical School and an internist at Cambridge Health Alliance, states "The current evidence does not convince me to recommend probiotics for any of my healthy patients." Nevertheless, probiotics are a $40 billion dollar industry. In the United States, most probiotics are sold as dietary supplements, which do not undergo the testing and approval process that drugs do.

Some studies suggest that certain probiotics can help in certain contexts. For example, Saccharomyces boulardii, a yeast, has been shown to reduce the risk of diarrhea in adults taking antibiotics. As you can see from this example, researchers have been able to identify a specific organism that seems to be beneficial. Even if you'd identified a microorganism that you thought might benefit you, the probiotic you purchase at a health food store may not contain the microorganisms listed on the label. Some university researchers used DNA analysis to compare the bacterial strains listed on the labels with the bacterial strains that actually resided in the product. They found that only one of the sixteen products they analyzed contained the strains listed on the label; some had entirely different bacterial species.

I've tried lots of probiotics and can't see that they've done anything for me. Considering that 99 percent of our gut bacteria are anaerobic (they function in an oxygen-free environment), and that probiotics are exposed to oxygen, it's not surprising that the probiotics we eat don't easily colonize our guts. In fact, they don't permanently colonize at all. Probiotics have been shown to be helpful in curing certain kinds of diarrhea, mostly in malnourished children. This may be because the one percent of gut bacteria that are aerobic live in the cecum, a cul-de-sac at the beginning of our large intestines where bacteria work on the partially digested food that become feces.

Overall, I agree with the notion that if you're a normal well-fed person, you don't need supplements. But there's still plenty of debate about this among researchers. Various studies show that some people may be deficient in certain vitamins or minerals. My husband and I and some friends have found that taking a supplement containing minerals such as calcium and magnesium has helped with leg cramps. I haven't taken them for a long time because the pills are too big. I also no longer get cramps but have no idea why.

The vast genetic variation among people may affect an individual's requirements for vitamins and minerals. For example: one man suddenly found that everything smelled and tasted either rotten or very strong. "All I could do was stand in the woods all day." He could eat only a few things, mostly cold and white. He went to doctor after doctor until finally one figured out his problem: his saliva had no zinc in it. He was cured with a prescription for zinc sulfate. This condition, by the way, is usually triggered by a bout of flu or a stay in the hospital. Go figure.

9. Body Weight

While I'd love to be thinner, I don't worry about being overweight—which I am, according to the BMI (body mass index) calculator. (BMI is a measure that uses your height and weight to work out if your weight is healthy—or so they say.) The easiest way to get your BMI is to use a calculator available on numerous internet sites. The definitions of what is "overweight," "normal," and "obese" are determined by the World Health Organization, National Heart, Lung and Blood Institute, and other organizations. They base their definitions on BMI figures as follows:

Underweight: Less than 18.5

Normal weight: 18.5 to 24.9

Overweight: 25 to 29.9

Obese: 30 or greater

At this writing, my BMI is 26.1—overweight. I'm not alone: 65 percent of my fellow Americans are also overweight, including Michael Jordan in his prime. The same was true for Arnold Schwarzenegger. When he was Mr. Universe at age thirty-three, Schwarzenegger had a

BMI of 33, which made him technically obese—and makes you question the BMI ratings. BMI measurements can't tell what percentage of your weight is from fat, muscle, or bone.

What's more, BMI does a poor job of predicting your metabolic health. In a 2016 study of more than 40,000 adults in the U.S., researchers compared people's BMIs with more specific measurements of their health, such as insulin resistance, triglycerides, inflammation, and glucose levels. Nearly half of those classified as overweight, and about a quarter of those classified as obese, were metabolically healthy by these measures. On the other hand, 31 percent of those with a "normal" body mass index were metabolically unhealthy.

Losing weight and keeping it off to achieve a "normal" BMI is next to impossible for most of us. Your body wants to be a certain weight, which is why you usually re-gain the weight you've lost by dieting. As I'm sure you've noticed, there's a weight you can maintain without any effort. That's the weight that your body fights to defend, whether you like it or not.

Dr. Rudy Liebel has devoted most of his career trying to determine the processes that regulate body fat. In carefully controlled studies, he sequestered volunteers who ranged from lean to obese in a hospital for months, rigorously controlling what they ate and how much they exercised. He altered their diets to make them gain and lose weight. Through it all, he took a wide array of measurements, including heart rate, muscle activity, energy expenditure, exhalation of carbon dioxide, metabolism of glucose, and much more. As he reports, "In all instances in which we have performed this experiment, which must number well over 40 now [late 1990s], the individuals fall back to their starting weight."

The system that regulates our weight is a highly complex one that keeps our weight within a narrow range. It's a feedback system that includes two centers in the brain, one that tells you if you're hungry and another that tells you you're full. It also includes fat cells, which release hormones that communicate with the brain, triggering the urge to eat or to stop eating. In other words, our fat cells maintain equilibrium between the forces that deposit fat and the forces that release fat. Neither eating less nor exercising more will lead to long-term weight loss because our bodies naturally compensate. As Sandra Aamodt, a neuroscientist, puts it, "The root of the problem [inability to lose weight and keep it off] is not willpower but neuroscience." When you lose weight, your brain declares a state of starvation emergency and institutes corrective measures. "The brain's weight-regulation system considers your set point to be the correct weight for you, whether or not your doctor agrees. Dieting is rarely effective, doesn't reliably improve health, and does more harm than good."

Here's an example that shows how our bodies fight to defend its fat: researchers studied the contestants on "The Biggest Loser" television show to see how they fared following their weight loss. Of the 14 contestants they studied, 13 regained most if not all their lost weight; four are heavier now than before the competition; only one, with great effort, has managed to maintain her weight. To make matters worse, the contestants' resting metabolisms became dramatically lower and stayed that way.

Dr. Kevin Hall, an expert on metabolism, spent more than ten years studying this phenomenon. He compared men and women who had lost large amounts of weight because of gastric bypass surgery with Big Bang contestants who had also lost large amounts of weight and who had continued to exercise to stave off muscle loss. Everyone's resting metabolic rate dropped, whether they remained well-muscled or not. In fact, the exercisers showed greater declines in resting metabolic rates than was the case for those who lost weight after bypass surgery. Basically, what happens is that, with drastic weight loss, your body senses starvation and reacts by lowering your metabolism. For the show contestants, exercising prompted their bodies to lower metabolism even more in an effort avoid starvation. After losing weight, their bodies were not burning enough calories to maintain their thinner weight. They had to eat even less. In addition, their fat cells increased the hormones that stimulated their hunger. The only way they could maintain their weight loss was to be hungry all the time. As one of the researchers said, "You can't get away from a basic biological reality. The body puts multiple mechanisms in place to get you back to your weight."

Other studies show the futility—and even the danger—of dieting. They show, for example, that 41 percent of dieters gain back more weight than they lose. In a study of 4,000 twins, researchers found that dieters were more likely to gain weight than their non-dieting identical twins. Even worse, studies show that dieters are more likely than non-dieters to become obese over the next one to 15 years. For example, a study of elite athletes who dieted to qualify for their weight classes (boxers and wrestlers) showed that they were three times more likely to be obese by age 60 than their peers who competed in other sports. Dr. Kevin Hall, PhD, at the National Institutes of Health, studies how the body responds to weight loss. His research helps to explain this phenomenon. For one thing, weight loss slows your metabolism—the breakdown of food and its transformation into energy—aka calorie burning. To make matters worse, our bodies prompt us to eat about 100 more calories than usual for every two pounds of weight loss. That is, the effect of appetite is three times stronger than the slowing metabolism. "It's this surge in appetite, even more than the drop in metabolism people have after weight loss, that drives weight regain," he says.

While it's true that our bodies want to maintain a certain weight, it's also true that it's common to gain weight as we get older. Speaking for myself and other women I know, I started gaining weight after menopause, a common occurrence for women. Most commonly, the weight is added to our midsections. One study showed that white women increased midsection fat by 24 percent. For Black women it was 17 percent. This belly fat accumulation is likely hormone related, but scientists don't know why it occurs. After losing a bit of my weight, I've stayed the same for about 25 years. Incidentally, you may have thought that metabolism begins to slow in middle age. The latest research shows that your metabolism holds steady until age 60, at which time it begins to decline at the rate of 0.7 percent a year.

Here's the good news: overweight people—as calculated by the BMI index—live longer than supposedly "normal" weight people. This has been well documented and is irrefutable. For example, a study that followed 1.8 million people for ten years found that people with a body mass index between 26 and 28 had the highest life expectancy. The study also showed that people with a BMI between 18 and 20 (supposedly optimal) had a lower life expectancy than those with a BMI between 34 and 36, which is categorized as obese. A study published in the May 2016 *Journal of the American Medical Association*, showed that people with a body mass index of 27 have the lowest risk of dying early from any cause. I have an acquaintance who is probably the fattest person I know. He is near 100 years old.

Another study, involving 250,000 people with heart disease found that overweight patients had better survival rates and fewer heart problems than those with a "normal" index number. Finally, in the study of the 90-plus-year-old residents of the retirement community that I mentioned in Chapter 3, the researchers found that people who were overweight or average weight outlived those who were underweight. As the lead researcher stated, "It turns out that the best thing to do as you age is to at least maintain or even gain weight."

By now, you may be convinced that our bodies want to maintain a certain level of fatness. Whether you're fat or thin, the system that regulates body weight is the same for all of us. That is, an obese person and a lean person both defend their body weights in the same way. As Dr. Liebel says, "When we study an obese person they really look metabolically just like a lean person, except they are bigger.... obese people require a larger mass of body fat to normalize their energy state."

I have always felt sympathetic toward fat people. They live in a world where most people see their obesity as a preventable problem: they eat too much; they don't exercise; they have no willpower. This is not true. The obese people I know eat carefully and exercise regularly. Incidentally, of the five or six obese people I know, only one has diabetes. Most of the diabetic people I know are thin.

Roxanne Gay, an obese woman, writes of her efforts to lose weight: "I am always trying to lose weight. I've tried Weight Watchers. I've tried low-carb diets. I've tried SlimFast during the day and one real meal at night. I've tried fasting every other day." To add to her misery, she must endure the scorn of others: "I am never allowed to forget the realities of my body, how my body offends the sensibilities of others, how my body dares to take up too much space. I hear the rude comments whispered. I see the stares and laughs and snickering. I see the thinly veiled or open disgust. People certainly try to shame me for being fat. When I am walking down the street, men lean out of their car windows and shout vulgar things at me about my body..."   Obese people like Ms. Gay do not lack willpower.   They're   merely   unlucky.   Evolutionary

Biologist Daniel Lieberman says, "When we blame people for being fat it's like blaming them for being human." Remember that.

To compound the problems of obese people, the medical establishment adds to their woes by shaming them. In an article in the *New England Journal of Medicine* titled "Our Culture of Shame," Dr. Scott Hagen laments the fact that "...weight bias remains common in health care settings and many practitioners accept the myth that obesity results primarily from lifestyle choices." In fact, in *The International Classification of Diseases*—the reference used for coding medical diagnoses—if you type in "obesity" you get "morbid (severe) obesity due to excess calories." Hagen's overweight patients expect scorn from him when they are unable to lose weight. Referring to one of his patients, who admits that he's "been bad lately," Dr. Hagen writes, "At every turn in my patient's experience with the health care system, well-intentioned clinicians would subject him to this idea"—that they lack discipline. "Messages about his weight were forced on him in every nook and cranny of his care, and any medical problem that could conceivably be related to his obesity was used as a weapon for counseling about doing more to lose weight." To make matters worse, health insurers can charge higher premiums for obese people: 25 to 50 percent more than coverage for people with a BMI below 30.

As to the world-wide rise in obesity, everyone seems to have an opinion about why this is so. Dr. Liebel's opinion is refreshing: "We simply do not know what environmental factors account for the increased prevalence of obesity."

10. Hydration

If I sweat a lot, I drink a lot. If not, I don't. I don't drink much plain water. I have nothing against it, but I prefer the taste of Chrystal Light when I get thirsty. It's a sugar-free lemonade. I hope it doesn't contain carcinogens.

The idea that you need to drink eight glasses of water a day was promulgated by the purveyors of bottled water, as I'll discuss below. There is absolutely no scientific evidence that drinking eight glasses of water a day has any health benefits, but it seems to be a persistent myth. In the words of Dr. Margaret McCartney in the *British Medical Journal*, it's "thoroughly debunked nonsense." My feelings exactly. (You may have heard that your urine color indicates our hydration status. There's no solid science behind that notion.)

Basically, your body will tell you when you need to drink something. As Dr. Aaron E. Carroll, professor of pediatrics at Indiana University School of Medicine, says, "the human body is finely tuned to signal you to drink long before you are actually dehydrated." Dr. Heinz Valtin, from Dartmouth University tells us that a large body of published experiments "attest to the precision and effectiveness of the osmoregulatory system for maintaining water balance" (i.e., if we need water, we get thirsty; if we have excess water, we get rid of it). Nephrologist Dr. Joel Topf agrees: most people aren't walking around chronically dehydrated and we don't need to be drinking water all day long.

And the drink needn't be water. It can be anything, including beer and coffee. A 2016 randomized controlled study concluded that the hydrating effects of water, coffee and tea were nearly identical. (The idea that coffee is a diuretic is also a myth.) Fruits and vegetables also contain a lot of water. In fact, in the U.S., 20 percent of the water we ingest comes from food.

As for "osmoregulation," the most important measure of hydration is the balance between electrolytes and water in your body. Electrolytes are nutrients/chemicals— including sodium, potassium, magnesium, and chlorine— that regulate nerve and muscle function, hydration levels, blood pH, blood pressure, and the rebuilding of damaged tissues. They are essential for life. When dissolved in water, electrolytes carry a charge. Our cells (especially nerve, heart, and muscle) use electrolytes to maintain voltages across their membranes, making it possible to carry nerve impulses and muscle contractions to other cells. For example, a muscle contraction needs calcium, sodium and potassium to contract properly. An imbalance can lead either to weak muscles, or muscles that contract too severely.

Your kidneys and several hormones normally keep electrolyte levels in balance. Your electrolyte levels tend to change when water levels in your body change. For example, when you become dehydrated, the concentration of electrolytes in your blood rises, which causes your body to release the hormone vasopressin, which in turn reduces the amount of water released into urine. In this way, water is conserved, and the balance is maintained. Drinking liquids restores your water level and your kidneys and hormones do the rest, again maintaining the balance.

Sometimes the level of an electrolyte in the blood can become too high or too low because of vomiting, diarrhea, kidney disease, cancer treatment, and some drugs, such as diuretics. (A study revealed that 20% of patients taking diuretics end up with reduced sodium and potassium levels.) Symptoms can include irregular heartbeat, weakness, twitching, confusion, seizures, and numbness. Most people who blame dehydration when they're feeling ill may actually be feeling ill because they're drinking *too much* water, according to one kidney function researcher. If you drink at a rate beyond what your kidneys can excrete, the electrolytes in your blood can become too diluted and make you feel "off."

As to drinks such as Gatorade that contain electrolytes, Tamara Hew-Butler, an exercise and sports scientist, says there's no scientific reason for most healthy people to drink beverages with added electrolytes unless you're doing intense exercise in the heat or otherwise losing lots of fluids. Most people get enough electrolytes from food, she says. On the other hand, as I can attest, Gatorade helps my husband ward off muscle cramps after golfing on hot days. When you exercise and sweat, you lose sodium and potassium. Dr. Ken Nosaka, Director of Exercise and Sports Science at Edith Cowan University (Australia), says 'Many people think dehydration causes muscle cramps and will drink pure water while exercising to prevent cramping. We found that people who solely drink plain water before and after exercise could in fact be making them more prone to cramps. This is likely because pure water dilutes the electrolyte concentration in our bodies and doesn't replace what is lost during sweating." Normally, however, you don't need to worry about electrolytes. Your body will keep them in balance.

Being dehydrated means not having enough water in your blood. If this happens, you get thirsty and you go for a drink, after which you're not thirsty anymore. But wait a minute! It takes ten or fifteen minutes for the water to make its way into your bloodstream. You certainly don't continue gulping water for ten minutes waiting for your thirst to be quenched. What stops you from continuing to drink water—which can actually be dangerous?

The answer: If we're like mice, on whom new research was conducted, we have cells in our brains that regulate thirst. But those cells don't respond to the water itself. They respond to the speed at which the water is ingested—that is, the gulps. In the mice, feeding them water-saturated gel or giving them sips didn't stimulate those cells. They would continue to drink even when they'd had enough. They needed those big swallows to quench their thirst. Regulating water in this way was surely an evolutionary benefit for us—it impels us to drink enough water to get to the next source, but not so much as to be life threatening. In addition to gulps, veins that carry nutrients and fluid into the liver are also involved in monitoring thirst. It's a complicated and not fully understood process, one that is so important to the body's functioning that our brains have multiple, redundant ways to monitor it.

Drinking too much water dilutes the blood, which throws off the sodium balance, which causes cells to swell. (The condition is called hyponatremia.) If the swelling occurs in the brain, you can die, as happened to several football players who overdid it. Since 2008 several high school football players are known to have died from drinking too much fluid during and after a practice. In cases like these, the body can't rid itself of the surplus water fast enough through sweating or urination. In trying to equalize sodium levels by drawing water from the blood and into the surrounding cells, the cells begin to swell. If this process occurs in the brain, it can be lethal.

When I do drink plain water, it comes from a tap and not from a plastic bottle. The bottled water industry is worth more than $15 billion annually. These companies keep the eight-glasses-of-water-myth alive by sponsoring "public service" messages and programs to promote more water drinking. For example, an initiative called Hydration for Health is sponsored by the manufacturers of Evian. Nestle sponsored a study that concluded that almost two-thirds of children in New York and Los Angeles weren't getting enough water. Ridiculous.

Here are some things you should know about bottled water:

- About half the people in the U.S. drink water from a bottle—either occasionally or as their main source—at the rate of 15 gallons per year.
- Twenty-five percent of the bottled water sold in the US comes from a municipal source (e.g., tap water).
- Half the leading bottled water brands get their water from drought-stricken California (my state).
- Fans of bottled water pay more than a 4,000 percent markup to buy a product that's virtually free.
- Drinking bottled water is a waste of your money. If you bought a single-serving bottle every day (about $1 apiece in New York), you'd spend about $365.
- Manufacturers use 17 million barrels of crude oil in their bottle production.
- On average, it takes 2,000 times more energy to bottle water, transport it, and refrigerate it than getting it from your tap.
- Global plastic consumption rose from 5.5 million tons in 1950 (when everyone got their water from a tap) to around 100 million tons in 2009.
- Just under a third of those billions of bottles sold in the U.S. is recycled.

As I said, when I drink water, it comes from a tap. I don't worry about it. But then, I don't live in Flint, Michigan.

11. Salt

I don't worry about eating too much salt. Sometimes I crave it, as I imagine most people do. I don't know whether the craving means my sodium level is down. Maybe it does, or maybe nobody knows. Salt (sodium) is one of the most important nutrients in your body. It maintains normal blood pressure, supports the work of nerves and muscles, and regulates your body's fluid balance. Your body strives to maintain a constant sodium level. If you have normal kidney function and blood pressure, your kidneys can deal with wide variations in sodium intake without increasing your blood pressure. For example, if you drink too much water or other liquids, your body excretes the excess water it doesn't need to maintain its sodium level.

Most Americans eat between 3.0 and 4.4 grams of salt per day, with women consuming less and men consuming more. (A teaspoon contains six grams of salt.) According to the USDA's Dietary Guidelines for Americans, that's too much. They recommend less than 2.3 grams a day, an amount that would supposedly lower blood pressure and, in turn, result in a lower incidence of cardiovascular disease. However, scientists reporting in the September 2021 issue of *Nutrients* found that current evidence indicates that "the risk of adverse health outcomes increases when sodium intake exceeds 5 g/day or is *below 3 g/day* [my italics]." In other words, the "sweet spot" for sodium intake is three to five grams a day, with "both lower and higher levels of intake associated with higher risk of cardiovascular disease or death." (The increased risk associated with five grams per day was largely confined to those with hypertension.) In studying populations worldwide, the scientists involved in this study found that, in fact, most people around the world consume this moderate range of salt (three to five grams a day)—a level "associated with the lowest risk of cardiovascular disease and mortality." What this study tells us is that you can ignore the Dietary Guidelines of 2.3 grams of salt per day.

In his clinic, Cardiologist Eric Topol finds a wide range of responses to salt intake. Some people are very sensitive to salt, in which case a small increase in salty foods can have a pronounced effect on their blood pressure. Others can eat salt-laden meals and their blood pressure will hardly budge. "Maybe," he says, "salt restriction really is beneficial for some, but we haven't defined the people yet that would drive that."

Interestingly, the notion that eating more salt makes us feel thirstier and impels us to drink more may be wrong. A meticulously conducted study of Russian cosmonauts held in isolation revealed that eating more salt made them *less* thirsty, a finding that contradicts much of the conventional wisdom about how our bodies handle salt. For the experiment, the cosmonauts were given varying amounts of salt, from a high of 12 grams daily, to a low of six grams daily. (Note that their "low" was significantly higher than the 2.3 grams recommended in the Dietary Guidelines.) The researchers measured the amount of sodium excreted in the crew's urine, the volume of their urine, and the amount of sodium in their blood. As they expected, the amount of sodium in the cosmonauts' blood remained constant. When they ate more salt, they excreted more salt and their urine volume increased.

What came as a surprise, after examining the cosmonauts' fluid intake, was the discovery that eating more salt didn't induce the cosmonauts to drink more liquids. In fact, the more salt the cosmonauts ate, the less fluids they drank. And yet, they were still excreting water. Where was that water coming from? It turns out that a high salt intake induced the cosmonauts' own bodies to generate the water. In this case, the water was a byproduct of the breakdown of fat and muscle in their bodies, similar to the way camels generate water: when traveling through the desert that has no water, the camels get water by breaking down the fat in their humps.

Oddly, the crew complained that they were always hungry on the high-salt diet, even though they were eating the same amount on the lower-salt diets, when hunger was not a problem. Not only were they hungrier, but they also lost weight! It turns out that the hunger and weight loss were the result of an increase in the production of glucocorticoid hormones, which influence both metabolism and immune function. (The scientists were careful to caution against eating salt to lose weight. They reason that more salt makes you hungrier in the long run and that high glucocorticoid levels are linked to such conditions as muscle loss, Type 2 diabetes, and other metabolic problems.)

Still, why do salty foods make us thirsty? Dr. Mark Zeidel, a nephrologist of Harvard Medical School, says that people and animals get thirsty because salt-detecting neurons in the mouth stimulate an urge to drink. This kind of thirst "may have nothing to do with the body's actual need for water." Apparently, scientists aren't sure about how salt affects us. Dr. Melanie Hoenig, an assistant professor of medicine at Harvard Medical School admits, "The work [the cosmonaut study] suggests that we really do not understand the effect of sodium chloride on the body."

What all of this says to me is not to worry about eating salt. We are probably eating the right amount. Besides, I think we can trust our bodies to deal with it.

12. Germs

One of my pet peeves is coming into a bathroom stall and seeing that the toilet seat is spattered with pee. This means that before sitting on the seat, I must take some toilet paper and wipe the seat until it's dry. Studies of toilet habits vary, but one study found that 85 percent of women said they crouched over public toilets, and 12 percent papered the seat. Only two percent sat all the way down. I'm one of the two percent. I'm not worried about germs on public toilet seats—or anywhere else, for that matter.

There's no reason to be afraid of germs on toilet seats. As Dr. William Schaffner, professor of preventive medicine at Vanderbilt University Medical Center says, "toilet seats are not a vehicle for the transmission of any infections agents—you won't catch anything." There's no medical evidence that anyone has ever picked up a venereal disease from a toilet seat. Any bacteria found on toilet seats are common skin microbes that we all carry around on our bodies. In fact, when studying bacteria on various surfaces in the bathroom, the toilet seat proved to be the cleanest surface.

Some experts define a sanitary surface as something clean enough to eat off of, with no more than 1,000 bacteria per square inch. On a 20/20 news program, Dr. Schaffner measured the bacteria on various surfaces, including those in a nearby bathroom as well as in the newsroom. He found that the toilet seat passed the sanitary test, but the anchorman's desk did not.

Dr. Chuck Gerba, professor of microbiology at the University of Arizona, measures bacteria in a variety of household objects. His studies found that the average toilet seat contains about 50 bacteria per square inch. "It's one of the cleanest things you'll run across in terms of micro-organisms. It's our gold standard—there are not many things cleaner than a toilet seat when it comes to germs."

So much for toilet seats. How about other surfaces? A sponge has about 10 million bacteria per square inch. I use sponges in the kitchen and elsewhere. I don't worry about germs on my sponges, especially given the fact that exposure to bacteria encourages a stronger immune system. A study of 1,037 children in New Zealand, which began in 1972 and continues to this day, showed that children who frequently sucked their thumbs or bit their nails (had their hands in their mouths) were significantly less likely to test positive for allergies than those who did not. Other studies have shown an increase in allergies and asthma in people living in overly sterile environments. Also, most people who use antibiotic soap are no healthier than those who use normal soap; and chronically sick people who use antibiotic soap appear to get sicker!

In March 1819, Dr. John Bostock reported the first case of hay fever—his own—to a medical society in London. More cases were soon reported. In looking into this new phenomenon, Bostock noted that the condition appeared only among the upper classes. "I have not heard of a single, unequivocal case occurring among the poor." It turned out that only the upper classes were affected because they had begun to clean up their environments. Cities in both the United States and United Kingdom had begun to institute major sanitary reforms. For the first time in human evolution, certain microbes and parasites were being removed from the human organism. Our bodies, which had evolved to work in concert with a vast and diverse array of microbes, would never work quite the same way again.

As one who doesn't believe in sanitizing everything—or, really, anything—I was heartened to read about an international project in which over 900 scientists and volunteers collected samples of microorganisms from subways in 60 cities and on six continents. They swabbed turnstiles, railings, ticket kiosks, benches, and subway cars. (One researcher was thanked by a bystander for cleaning the subway.) They found 4,246 *known* species of micro-organisms. Two thirds of these were bacteria and the remainder were a mix of fungi, viruses, and other kinds of microbes. They also found 10,928 viruses and 748 kinds of bacteria that had *never been documented*. The vast majority of the collected organisms pose little risk to humans. As one scientist reported, "We don't see anything that we are worried about. People are in contact with these all the time." In fact, nearly all of the new viruses the researchers found are likely to be bacteriophages—viruses that infect bacteria. Half of the bacteria the researchers identified were those that typically live in and on the human body, especially the skin. Some of the bacteria included those that live in soil. They also found a species typically associated with the ocean. All this is to say that microbes are a natural part of our environment. You can't avoid the little creatures and you can't get rid of them.

In the interests of science, I sent swabs of my skin to American Gut, a non-profit research group that studies people's microbiomes—mostly the gut stuff. (Your *microbiome* consists of the microorganisms, such as bacteria, viruses, and fungi that inhabit your body.) I was astonished to get back a list of *276 different genera* of bacteria living on my hand, which could amount to thousands of different species. (If you remember your biology, animal taxonomy goes in the following order: kingdom, phylum, class, order, family, genus, species. The lab results drilled down only as far as genera, the plural word for genus). I learned that the second-most predominant genus of bacteria on my hand is Streptococcus—a genus that includes the species responsible for necrotizing fasciitis (flesh-eating bacteria)! Happily, the Streptococcus genus also includes bacteria that form mutually beneficial relationships with other bacteria. Even better, scientists have discovered a strain of *Staphylococcus epidermis* that produces a chemical that kills several types of cancer cells. As Richard Gallo,

Distinguished Professor and the Founding Chairman of the Department of Dermatology at the University of California, San Diego, tells us, "...the skin microbiome is an important element of human health. In fact, we previously reported that some bacteria on our skin produce antimicrobial peptides that defend against pathogenic bacteria such as Staph aureus."

Handwipes, such as you see at supermarkets for wiping the handles of shopping carts, do more harm than good. They disrupt the natural balance of bacteria on our hands. These wipes, and many other products, are impregnated with a chemical called *triclosan*, which kills the native bacteria on our hands, some of which protect us from invaders. Even worse, triclosan kills weak bacteria but favors those that can tolerate the chemical, including those that eat triclosan! In other words, overuse of such products helps encourage antibiotic-resistant germs. Not only that, but triclosan has entered our water system where it has been found to disrupt the endocrine systems of fish, the result of which is lower sperm counts than in fish that are not exposed to triclosan.

As shown by my hand analysis, 90 percent of the cells on your body are not your own. They belong to the more than 100 trillion microorganisms—such as bacteria, viruses and fungi—that live in your gut, mouth, skin and everywhere else. In fact, you're carrying around about three pounds of these organisms. Your gut alone contains about 40,000 species of bacteria. For every one of your own genes you have 100 genes from the microorganisms. We pick up the organisms that make up our microbiomes at birth with our trip through the birth canal. From that point on, we are "seeded" with microorganisms through our continuing contact with our home environment.

It's kind of a creepy idea, but microbes help you digest food, synthesize essential nutrients and vitamins, and prevent disease-causing pathogens from invading your body. Substances must first pass through layers of microbiota on the skin, gut, and airways at which point they may be sequestered, excluded, or metabolized before they enter our cells. At the same time, the microbiota are busy training our immune systems to recognize unwanted invaders.

Scientists are now looking at the ways in which our health has been affected by changes to our microbiomes over the last 75 years—changes brought about by modern sanitation, water treatment, and medical practices, including the overuse of antibiotics. Such practices have reduced species diversity within our bodies—species with which we co-evolved millions of years ago. Our immune systems evolved to anticipate the bacteria, worms, and other organisms commonly found in vegetation, mud and water throughout evolution. Because we are less exposed to microbes than in the past, our immune systems are not being challenged in the ways they once were. Some scientists have suggested that the reduction of diversity account for the rise in diseases such as diabetes, heart disease, asthma, autism, inflammatory bowel disease, obesity, and many more. Many—if not most—of these diseases were virtually unknown 75 years ago. For example, a bacterium called *Heliobacter pylori* once occupied the stomach of nearly every person in the world, having been intertwined with our species for at least two hundred thousand years. Now it is found in just five percent of children born in the United States. *H. pylori* plays a role in regulating stomach acid and in quieting the inflammatory response. While it can cause ulcers, the near eradication of this bacterium has now been shown to have a serious downside. Many Americans now suffer from acid reflux, and the rate of a certain type of esophageal cancer has soared. What's more, researchers have found the lack of *H. pylori* to be implicated in the rise of asthma and allergies.

More than 60 percent of human infectious diseases are zoonotic—that is, they're the result of humans coming into contact with a virus-carrying animal. The virus takes advantage of the new host and colonizes it. Such is the case with the virus that causes Covid-19 as well as the one that causes AIDS. While the viruses that cause Covid-19 and AIDS are quite successful in their ability to infect people, the most successful of the zoonotic viruses is the Epstein-Barr virus (EBV), a very transmissible species of herpesvirus that may reside within at least 90 percent of us, including me and half of five-year-old children.

EBV is passed from person to person through bodily fluids, mostly saliva. With most of us, when we become infected we don't get particularly sick and we develop immunity. The virus remains inactive within our bodies for the rest of our lives. If infection doesn't occur until we're adolescents, we have about a fifty percent chance of getting mononucleosis.

But it's not all that benign. EBV has been implicated in a bunch of diseases, especially autoimmune diseases such as lupus, multiple sclerosis, and rheumatoid arthritis. But it's also been implicated in other diseases, including Parkinson's disease, schizophrenia, and a whole bunch of cancers. It's actually a rather long list. Some researchers theorize that the symptoms of long-haul Covid are caused by the coronavirus reactivating dormant Epstein-Barr virus. Too late to start worrying about that one.

At the beginning of the Covid-19 pandemic, I was careful not to touch the handrail at the post office. When I got home, I washed my hands. I only followed this regimen one time. I just couldn't get into it, mostly because I'm not a fearful person but also because the rate of infection in our area was low. (I also bought no bleach or hand sanitizer.) Lucky for me, researchers have now learned that the risk of Covid-19 infection by touching contaminated surfaces is also low: a 1 in 10,000 chance.

Nevertheless, people continued to sanitize everything, which is probably not a good thing. Some health experts fear that many of the sanitizing efforts, if they continue, may pose a threat to human health. The problem is that excessive hygiene practices—including social distancing and inappropriate antibiotic use—will negatively affect our microbiome. As one researcher remarked, "We're starting to realize that there's collateral damage when we get rid of good microbes, and that has major consequences for our health." The consequences include promoting sickness and imperiling out immune systems. Bacteria train our immune systems and produce molecules that affect the workings of every cell and organ in our bodies, including our brains, spinal cords, and joints. All of this supports what is called the "hygiene hypothesis" which holds that our germaphobic ways may be making us sick by harming our microbiome. We end up with an underutilized immune system unable to distinguish friend from foe.

As for viruses, as nasty as some can be, we can't live without them. Living within us are types of viruses called *phages*, meaning bacteria eaters. Our bodies are home to trillions of them. So far, scientists have identified 21,000 species of phages living in our guts. Most of them infect the bacteria, fungi, and other single-celled organisms that live inside us. Some studies suggest that our resident viruses help keep our bodies in balance, preventing any one species from getting out of control and making us sick. Remnants of a virus that invaded our shrew-like ancestors more than 100 million years ago live within us today. In other words, the DNA of viruses are part of our own DNA. Today we carry about a hundred thousand fragments of viral DNA, which make up eight percent of the human genome. Viruses—they are us.

Even though I don't worry about germs and believe that some sanitation practices do more harm than good, I certainly would not want to return to a time or live in a place where no sanitation programs had been instituted—times and places, for example, where raw sewage runs in the streets. We're clearly better off having sewers, vaccines, and antibiotics. Still, we must be aware of the price we're paying for these advances and take steps to curtail them whenever their effects have been shown to do more harm than good.

13. Skin

My skin is rather awful, mostly because it's covered in little crusty patches called actinic keratosis. You may have a few of them, too. Many people have them removed. Supposedly, they can become cancerous, but that has never been the case with me. In fact, it's quite rare. I don't worry about them and mostly ignore them. The fact that I'm riddled with these things is kind of mysterious. Although they're supposedly a result of sun damage, I have them in places "where the sun don't shine," including the base of my thumb (palm side), the inside of my forearm, and groin. My dermatologist says "genetic." But my parents didn't have these. Neither does my sister or my sixty-year-plus kids. Incidentally, even though I see a dermatologist every now and then, I don't have annual skin checks and have never had a full-body skin check. When offered, I always turn them down. So far, so good.

In addition to actinic keratosis, I've also had basal cell skin cancers, but no melanoma (the serious kind). Even so, I don't use sunscreen. (Neither does my husband, who has had no skin cancer.) I don't use sunscreen mostly because of the bother, but also because I figure it's too late. Most of the damage has been done. Maybe it's just as well: I learned that sunscreen products commonly include a chemical called nano-titanium dioxide (TiO2), a product that kills good bacteria on your skin. The good bacteria include a common strain of *Staphylococcus epidermis*. You don't want to kill these bacteria. Richard Gallo, Distinguished Professor and the Founding Chairman of the Department of Dermatology at the University of California, San Diego, tells us that "This unique strain of skin bacteria produces a chemical that kills several types of cancer cells but does not appear to be toxic to normal cells." So—sunscreens kill bacteria that kill cancer. "There is increasing evidence," Gallo says, "that the skin microbiome is an important element of human health. In fact, we previously reported that some bacteria on our skin produce antimicrobial peptides that defend against pathogenic bacteria such as Staph aureus."

Perhaps not all sunscreens contain nano-titanium dioxide, but you can't tell which have the chemical and which don't. According to the National Institutes of Health, sunscreen producers are not required to list the ingredients. Thus, they report, consumers "…are unable to switch to an alternative because it is unknown to them which alternative does not contain the experimental material." Because sunscreen ingredients are not labeled, The NIH calls the use of TiO2-containing sunscreens a "societal experiment." (Incidentally, the International Agency of Research on Cancer has categorized TiO2 as a potential human carcinogen.) At least I'm not an unwitting participant in an experiment.

Sunscreens are one of the 100,000 drugs on the market that have not been reviewed by the FDA—that is, have not been deemed to be safe and effective. Beginning in 1997, scientists discovered that oxybenzone, the chemical that filters out UV rays, does not stay on the surface of the skin but is absorbed. It has been found in urine and breast milk. The CDC found that 97 percent of sunscreen-users' urine samples contained the chemical. At the same time, there's never been any indication that sunscreen chemicals are harmful to humans, and evidence has shown that sunscreen can prevent skin cancer. Still, because sunscreens have not been studied, we don't know about long-term effects.

As I'm sure you're aware, our microbiome—the bacteria, viruses, fungi, etc., that inhabit our bodies—has become a popular area of study. Until recently, the technology required to sequence the DNA of all these microbes wasn't available. Now that it is, scientists are learning more and more about the importance of these microbes to our health—including that of our skin. As you might remember from high school biology, skin is the body's largest organ. If you laid it out, it would cover around twenty square feet. On those twenty square feet, we harbor around a billion bacteria per centimeter. The bacteria species vary according to the skin environment: oily (forehead and chest); moist (armpits and creases in our elbows, knees and groin); and dry (forearms, stomach, chest, etc.) The highest bacterial biomass is our armpits. It's the reason people use deodorants.

Scientists, such as Dr. Jack Gilbert and Dr. Julie Segre, who study microbial ecosystems and the human genome, remind us that most of our skin microbes are important to the skin's function and thus to the functioning of our immune systems. Removing microbes from our skin opens up space for more microbes—including pathogens—to take refuge. For this reason, it's become popular in certain circles to avoid using soap when washing. Some people avoid washing altogether. A few years ago, I quit using soap on my face and most of the rest of my body. I don't want to mess up my microbiome. In studying this topic, however, I learned that it's difficult to permanently change the basic skin microbiome of an adult. Because the skin microbiome comes from deep in our pores, even if we remove the bacteria, our skin repopulates with the microbiome that was established in infancy. So maybe we shouldn't worry about washing off our skin bacteria. Still, I'm sticking with my regimen—leaving my microbiome alone as much as possible.

As to my skin cancers, they're not the serious kind. Here's a little primer on skin cancer:

- **Actinic keratosis**: a patch of thick, scaly, or crusty skin. Though they are considered pre-cancerous, less than one percent develop into squamous cell cancers per year (per person). The usual treatment for actinic keratosis is to freeze them off with liquid nitrogen.

- **Basal cell carcinoma**: the most common kind of cancer in humans. Basal cell carcinoma is simply cancer of the basal cells in the skin—the cells in the lowest layer of the epidermis. They grow slowly, and usually do not metastasize.

- **Squamous cell carcinoma**: like basal cell carcinomas, they are cancers of a layer of skin cells—the squamous cells. Squamous cell cancers are more likely to grow into deeper layers of skin and spread to other parts of the body than basal cell cancers, although this is uncommon. At any rate, they're considered more dangerous than basal cell carcinomas.

- **Melanoma cancers**: develop from melanocytes, the pigment-making cells of the skin. Melanomas are much less common than basal and squamous cell cancers, but they are more likely to grow, metastasize, even kill you if untreated. You'd do well to be aware of new spots on your skin or spots that are changing in size, shape or color and that are asymmetrical, with irregular edges and a color that is not uniform.

I've found all my basal cell cancers myself. They feel like little bumps under the surface of my skin (face and neck). Because they're not visible on the surface, I've always had to point them out to my dermatologist, who biopsies them. I asked her about ignoring them. She said she thinks about this and has decided that if it looks like you've got five years of life left in you, you should have them removed. For all I know, if I hadn't found the cancers myself, they might still be there, still invisible and causing no problem.

My first skin cancer treatment was probably 30 years ago. It was for a basal cell carcinoma on my nose. After confirming the diagnosis, my dermatologist at the time sent me to a plastic surgeon to have it removed. After removal, however, an examination of the tissue showed that the edges were not clean. In other words, they had not gotten it all. So I had radiation on my nose—two weeks of daily treatments, as I recall. Incidentally, this dermatologist mentioned a treatment called Mohs surgery but said he didn't know how to do this. Then he warned me that, should I find someone who would use the Mohs procedure, I might end up with a big nostril. That was the last time I went to that dermatologist, who now regularly performs Mohs surgeries.

The Mohs technique, which is named after Dr. Frederic Mohs, is one in which the doctor removes little bits at a time, checking the bits under a microscope between each removal while you wait. This process continues until the edges are clean. In this way, the surgeon removes just what's necessary. I now have an excellent dermatological surgeon who has used the Mohs technique to remove four basal cell cancers on my face and neck.

Because Mohs surgery is more expensive than other techniques and highly profitable, some say the surgery is overused. For example, if the cancer is on a place where scarring is not an issue, it's cheaper to just cut off a larger slice in the initial incision and be done with it. As of 2014, the incidence of Mohs surgery increased by more than 400 percent in 10 years, which may be due in part because of our aging population.

If I find another one of those invisible bumps, I've decided to ignore it and not worry about it.

14. Joint and Back Pain

I have arthritis in my knees. When I started writing this book, at age 85, I had pain in my knees, but it was manageable. Walking on level ground wasn't especially painful. I didn't consider knee replacements. As time went on, however, my knees got worse and one began to swell. As I write this paragraph, I'm recovering from replacements on both knees. So far, so good.

One thing I never considered was arthroscopic surgery. I'd read that this surgery was useless. In arthroscopic surgery, a procedure that was started in the 1970s, the surgeon makes a couple of small incisions in the knee and inserts a fiber-optic arthroscope to look around, then washes out the joint with about ten quarts of saltwater to remove bits of cartilage, bony fragments, calcium crystals, and inflammatory cells. He or she may also smooth out frayed cartilage and meniscus that cover the top and sides of the knee. It sounds like it should be helpful, but it's not.

By 2002, fourteen studies had shown that arthroscopic surgery offered substantial pain relief. None, however, compared people who had had the arthroscopic surgery with those who hadn't. In 2002, researchers at the Houston Veterans Affairs Medical Center and Baylor College of Medicine attempted to make this comparison using three groups of patients—180 in all. Two thirds had arthroscopic surgery, either just the washing or the cartilage cleanup. One third had a sham surgery—small incisions in the knee, but nothing else. In this latter case, the medical team acted as though they were performing all the treatments. For this experiment, one surgeon, the orthopedic surgeon for an NBA team, performed all the procedures.

During the next two years the patients were evaluated for knee pain and function. It turns out, there was no difference in outcome between those who had the procedure and those who had not. As reported in the *New England Journal of Medicine*, editors wrote, "Although smoothing cartilage and meniscal irregularities may sound appealing, larger forces within and outside the joint environment, such as malalignment, muscle weakness, instability, and obesity, which are not addressed by this type of surgery, may have greater effects on the clinical outcome...[the procedures] may simply remove some of the evidence while the destructive forces continue to work."

Since then, according to my source, Dr. Paul Offit, "...fourteen randomized, controlled clinical trials and twelve observational studies, involving 1.8 million people, found that arthroscopic surgery for knee arthritis, with or without repair of a torn meniscus, was no better than physical therapy alone. Arthroscopic surgery, therefore, is

115

no longer recommended for the treatment of knee arthritis. Yet, it remains one of America's most common outpatient surgical procedures."

As to tears in the meniscus, at least five different high-quality randomized controlled trials show that meniscus surgery is also next to useless. Nevertheless, every year about 400,000 middle-aged and older Americans have the surgery. The thing is, there is no clear relationship between knee pain and meniscus tears. In fact, most people over forty have a meniscus tear and most do not have pain. When people undergo the surgery and report feeling better, the result is probably due to the placebo effect.

Bad knees can get better without surgery. For one thing, new studies have shown that humans can re-grow cartilage—rather like a salamander does when it re-grows missing limbs. The science has to do with the production of new collagen proteins and is rather complicated. At any rate, as one researcher said, "...this study provides compelling evidence that there are many similarities in human and salamander limbs." Richard Bedard, author of *Saving My Knees,* was told by four different doctors that his bad knees would never get better. He was in his 40s. He wouldn't take no for an answer and began a "research odyssey." He found several studies that proved that cartilage can indeed regrow, as shown in "before" and "after" MRI images. He started a program to heal his knees, which he reveals in his book. (I haven't read it., so I can't tell you the methods he used.) His conclusion: "My own experience showed me that rehabilitating damaged cartilage is a long, trying process. The condition of this tissue changes very, very slowly. But change it does—both better and worse. Today, after a recovery that took almost two years, my knees feel fine."

If your arthritis is bad and continues to be painful no matter what you try, you can opt for knee replacement surgery, which has a ten-year success rate of more than 90 percent. The same goes for hip replacement surgery. In joint replacement surgeries, the surgeon removes the damaged parts and replaces them with artificial parts. Almost one million hip and knee replacement surgeries are performed in the United States annually, and its success is worth noting.

Joint replacement surgery is lucrative business for device makers. An artificial hip costs about $350 to manufacture. But hospitals pay an average $4,500 to $8,000 for the device. In the case of one manufacturer, Medtronic, the overall cost of making its products is about 25 percent of what it sells them for, yielding a gross profit margin of about 75 percent. After purchasing the device, the hospital then marks up the price for sale to the patient. Plus, there are the kickbacks. That is, device manufacturers pay doctors to use their products. In 2007, the five major device manufacturers paid over $200 million to about five hundred orthopedic surgeons. As for the cost to you (or your insurance provider), the cost of implant procedures varies according to where you live. Overall, the cost averages $30,000. It's cheapest in Birmingham, Alabama ($11,327) and highest in Boston ($73,987)—a significant cost variation.

In the course of my research, I've learned that you need to be wary of medical devices, which, in addition to artificial joints, include pacemakers, stents, surgical mesh, vein filters, insulin pumps and the like. To increase sales, device makers strive to constantly innovate. After a manufacturer has updated a device, they can get it quickly to market because of the FDA's fast-track process—known as a 510(k), which exempts products from full review if they are "substantially equivalent" to ones already on the market. Manufacturers are not required to submit clinical data that demonstrate safety and effectiveness. As a result, untested devices come onto the market.

Not only that, but, unlike Canada, Australia, Japan, New Zealand and several European countries, the U.S. has no registry of implants that would provide the FDA, doctors, and patients with information about the risks and benefits of implants over time. Repeated efforts to implement a registry system in the U.S. have failed, thanks to the implant industries' powerful lobby. Even though there's no registry, in 2015 the FDA received around sixteen thousand reports of deaths associated with medical devices. But the number is surely higher: 99 percent of "adverse events" are not reported. The more serious the event, the less likely it is to be reported. The true number of those deaths could be as high as 1.6 million, making them one of the leading causes of death in the U.S. About 1,100 of these devices are recalled annually. For example, in 2013, 33,000 inferior vena cava filters were recalled. Instead of stopping blood clots from reaching the heart, the filters actually caused clots to form.

Back pain is another condition that plagues Americans—65 million people. In fact, low back pain is the number one cause of disability throughout the world. More than 1,500,000 opt for back operations each year. The record of success is pretty dismal. One study looked at the records of 1,450 patients diagnosed with disc problems. Half had two or more vertebrae fused; the other half had no surgery. After two years, only 26 percent of those who had the surgery returned to work while 67 percent who'd not had surgery returned to work. Unsurprisingly, 41 percent of those who'd had the surgery increased their use of opiates.

Complicated spine surgeries that involve fusing two or more vertebrae are on the rise. Between 1995 and 2010, there was an eight-fold jump in this type of operation. For some patients, there is a legitimate need for spine surgery and fusion, says Dr. Charles Burton, medical director for The Center for Restorative Spine Surgery in St. Paul, Minn. "But the concern is that it's gotten way beyond what is reasonable or necessary. There are some areas of the country where the rate of spine surgery is three or four times the national average."

Dr. William Welch, chief of neurosurgery at Pennsylvania Hospital, admits "We are less successful at treating back pain" than leg pain. The reason, Welch says, is that it's often hard to pinpoint the exact cause of someone's back pain. Even MRIs can be misleading because abnormalities, such as degenerating discs, *can be seen on scans for virtually everyone over the age of 30 regardless of whether they have pain.* [italics mine]" In other words, we all have degenerating disks.

One of my sources for useless surgeries is Ian Harris, MD, PhD—an Australian orthopedic surgeon and professor of orthopedic surgery who directs a research unit that focuses on surgical outcomes. He admits to performing surgery that doesn't work. Sometimes, he says, "If a patient complains enough, one of the easiest ways of satisfying them is to operate." The title of his book, by the way, is *Surgery, the Ultimate Placebo.* If we expect a treatment to work, it is more likely to be perceived as working.

In addition to designating spinal fusion and arthroscopy as being useless surgeries, Dr. Harris includes vertebroplasty/kyphoplasty (injecting a sort of cement into the spine to shore it up); coronary stenting (placing a tube inside an artery to open it up); shoulder surgery for impingement; ruptured Achilles' tendon surgery (wearing a boot works just as well); and many fracture surgeries (if the bones are roughly aligned, they will heal themselves).

Dr. David Kallmes of the Mayo Clinic believes that doctors continue to do some of these operations because insurers pay and because doctors remember their patients who seemed better afterward. "I think there is a placebo effect not only on patients but on doctors."

Now, it turns out, taking steroids or anti-inflammatory drugs, such as Advil and Aleve, increases your chances of developing chronic pain in your lower back, as reported in *Science Translational Medicine* (2022). Anti-inflammatories offer relief from acute pain, but because they inhibit inflammation, healing is also inhibited.

120

Inflammation is a normal part of recovering from an injury. Researchers discovered that people whose low back pain did resolve had high inflammation driven by neutrophils, a type of white blood cell that helps the body fight infection, the study said. As one of the researchers remarked, "Neutrophils dominate the early stages of inflammation and set the stage for repair of tissue damage. Inflammation occurs for a reason, and it looks like it's dangerous to interfere with it."

Recurring back pain often creates what researchers call "spiral of decline:" You take to your bed or couch because of the pain. This inactivity weakens muscles and joints, leaving your back and core even more feeble which then leads to more pain and more inactivity—and so on. One study of back pain, published in *JAMA Internal Medicine*, began by looking at 6,000 previously published studies on the topic of back pain prevention. Of this number, they found only 23 studies that they considered to be reliable. Those 23 studies looked at 30,000 people with back pain and the techniques used to treat them. The techniques included education about lifestyle changes, shoe orthotics, back belts, various types of exercise programs, and exercise programs that also included some type of education about back pain prevention.

Here's what they found: educational efforts alone, back belts, and orthotics were almost completely ineffective. But exercise programs, either with or without an educational element, proved to be effective in preventing recurrences of back pain. In fact, according to one researcher, "the size of the protective effect" from exercise

121

"was quite large." Exercise combined with education reduced the risk of an episode of low back pain in the next year by 45 percent. "Of all the options currently available to prevent back pain, exercise is really the only one with any evidence that it works."

The type of exercise program didn't matter: some regimens focused on strengthening muscles in the core and back; others combined aerobic conditioning with strength and balance training. But here's the rub: stopping the exercise regimen will also halt its protective effects.

A technique called "mindfulness-based stress reduction" also works for some people. It's a combination of meditation, body awareness and yoga. It focuses on increasing awareness and acceptance of one's experiences, whether they involve physical discomfort or emotional pain.

Exercise and stress reduction for low back pain supports the ideas of Dr. John E. Sarno (1923-2017). Dr. Sarno was a rehabilitation-medicine specialist at New York University who had an unconventional approach for dealing with back pain that made him the laughingstock among his peers. Because he had been seeing a therapist to determine whether his own ailments might have a psychological component, he started asking his patients about their histories. He discovered that his patients' psychic health was a major contributor to their pain. Except in rare cases, he believed, back pain has no structural basis. Instead, it is caused by feelings, such as anxiety or anger, that you unconsciously shift to the muscles in your lower back, which begin to spasm. The spasms lead to fear, and then more spasms, and eventually a vicious cycle of pain.

Sam Dolnick, the assistant managing editor of *The New York Times*, wrote a tribute to Sarno in the *Times Magazine* in which he describes Sarno's belief that "...the body was using physical pain to defend itself from mental anguish....Your back doesn't hurt because you lifted that heavy suitcase; your back hurts because you're smoldering with unacknowledged rage that your sister, who always got away with everything, still hasn't repaid that loan you couldn't afford to give her in the first place."

Dolnick is a believer: "Some 15 years ago, when I was in my 20s, I had terrible back pain, and an eminent doctor recommended that I have spinal surgery. On a relative's recommendation, I went to see Sarno for a second opinion. Limping into his office, I found a tiny, owlish man sitting behind a giant wooden desk. ...He asked why I had come to see him, and I described my problems with my back and then with my life. He was kind and inquisitive but firm. He had seen people like me before. There's nothing wrong with you, he said. Don't have surgery. Stop acting sick. Your back is fine, and so are you. He gave me his book [*Healing Back Pain*], and I watched his videos (they have the distinct feel of public-access TV), but mostly I tried to stop treating myself like an invalid. I threw away the back braces, started playing basketball again and watched, amazed, as the pain gradually went away. I can't say that I quite understand what happened with my back, but Sarno believed that I was suppressing a white-hot anger I could not articulate. Anger was always the most powerful emotion in Sarno's cosmology, the root cause of the physical pain."

Because I don't have problems with back pain, I can't add a testimony. But Sarno had plenty of admirers, including Howard Stern, who dedicated his book to Sarno. You can read testimonials on the webpage *thankyoudrsarno.com*. They're quite interesting.

Of course, when people opt for surgeries, they're looking for pain relief—a target also aimed at by pharmaceutical companies. They're knocking themselves out trying to find new pain relievers. So far, they aren't having much luck. Pain is complicated and not fully understood. Bear in mind that pain is a crucial survival mechanism. It keeps us from harming ourselves, which is what happens to people with the genetic abnormality called congenital insensitivity to pain (CIP). In this case, pain-sensing neurons are ineffective. Case in point: word got out to pain researchers that a boy from Pakistan was entertaining tourists by sticking knives through his arms and walking across burning coals. Before the researchers could study him, he'd jumped off a building and died. He might have felt no pain, but he was not immune to death.

At the opposite end of the pain spectrum, beginning with feeling no pain, is the "man on fire" syndrome: searing, excruciating, pain in response to mild warmth—as mild as walking into a 68-degree room. In this case, the pain-sensing neurons are hyperactive. These extreme cases—insensitivity and hyperactivity—are variations of the ordinary pain we all experience when we're injured or sick: the pain is caused by the activation of peripheral neurons that send their pain signals up our spinal cords and into our brains. This type of pain falls into the *acute* category and is what sends us to doctors.

The other category is *persistent* pain, characterized by chronic burning, deep aching, and electric shock-like sensations. Its mechanism is completely different from acute pain and is caused by cells in the brain called glia, which function as a kind of glue to hold neurons in place, but which also, as scientists have recently learned, supply them with nutrients and oxygen, insulate one neuron from another, and destroy pathogens. Unfortunately, they also promote an exaggerated pain response by enhancing neuronal firing when stimulated by a variety of triggers, such as a protein sent from sensory neurons following an injury. They're also triggered by immune cells sent to the brain by the central nervous system's lymphatic system. Researchers are now recognizing that glial cells are probably implicated in inflammatory diseases such as rheumatoid arthritis and osteoarthritis. They've also discovered that women are more prone to persistent pain than men, but they haven't figured out why. Finally, they've found that opioid drugs are not useful—and can be harmful—in persistent pain. As my source, *The Scientist* online magazine says, "...persistent pain is a very complex, multicellular disease state." So far, there's not much on the horizon in the way of help.

As for myself, I've found that injections of cortisone shots in my joints have been helpful, but probably a mistake. Cortisone reduces inflammation, swelling, and pain. But the shots don't otherwise fix anything. I've had four or five injections over the years, a couple of times in my hips for bursitis, and a few times in my knees because of pain and swelling. In a couple of cases, I've found the pain relief to be permanent, but usually the shots' effects last only three or four weeks. You shouldn't get too many cortisone shots over a short period of time. They can damage the tendons, ligaments, and cartilage. If you notice that pain relief from cortisone shots becomes shorter and shorter over time, it's not because you've built up a tolerance but because your joint is degrading. We can't stop the degradation, but by strengthening surrounding muscles and keeping active we can mitigate the effects.

15. Sleep

I never get eight hours of sleep. I usually sleep between six and seven hours a night—and my sleep is often interrupted. I don't worry about it. I figure my body will get the sleep it needs. I'd prefer not to have interrupted sleep—lying there in the dark for one or two hours is boring. On the other hand, it's a good time for thinking. I've done some good problem solving and have come up with creative ideas in the middle of the night. What's more, on those nights when I get less than six hours of sleep, I never feel the effects the next day.

I've always thought the notion that everyone needs eight hours of sleep a night was hogwash. This type of admonition just worries people and drives them toward medications. "Experts" say that sleeping less than seven hours per night on a regular basis is associated with adverse outcomes, such as diabetes, heart disease, hypertension, and a lot more. I don't buy that either. As it turns out, now scientists are saying some people do well on less sleep. As far as I'm concerned, this is a no-brainer, especially when you look at those who sleep far less than eight hours a night: Thomas Edison (three or four hours); President Clinton (five to six hours); Martha Stewart (four to five hours); Jay Leno (five hours).

My sleep pattern is normal. It turns out that the "lie down and die" model of sleep, in which we attempt to lie perfectly still for a solid eight-hour block, is a relatively new model that coincides with the industrial age. Like me, pre-industrial people experienced a "broken" pattern, splitting their slumber into "first" and "second" periods. Kroger Ekrich, author of *At Day's Close: Night in Times Past,* says "there is every reason to believe that segmented sleep, such as many wild animals exhibit, had long been the natural pattern of our slumber before the modern age, with a provenance as old as humankind."

When you look at the conditions under which humans evolved, it doesn't make sense that they'd basically go unconscious for eight hours in a row. There were too many pressures and predators to contend with. Some non-Western peoples, such as the !Kung hunter-gatherers in Africa or Balinese farmers in Indonesia have no specific bedtimes. Rather, they drift in and out of slumber depending on what's happening on any given night.

Researchers have also studied the sleep habits of three hunter-gatherer societies, two in Africa (the Hadza and San tribes) and one in Bolivia (the Tismane people). These tribes live much as their ancestors have for tens of thousands of years. By studying these people, the researchers could determine how early humans were "programmed" to sleep, and, by extension, what normal sleep might be for us. Like early humans, the hunter-gatherer people sleep outside or in crude huts and their only light at night comes from fire. What the researchers found is that, on a typical night, these people sleep slightly less than the average American. In the U.S., most adults sleep seven hours or more a night—although many sleep significantly less. Members of these hunter-gatherer tribes slept just *six and a half hours*. Researchers also found that the presence or absence of daylight is not the primary factor in their sleep patterns.

The conventional thinking has been that the artificial light throws off our biological clocks and if we could live like early humans, going to bed when the sun goes down and getting up when the sun comes up, we'd be much better off. It turns out that the people in all three of these tribes do not follow that sundown/sunup scenario. Instead, they stay awake several hours after the sun goes down and do not wake at sunrise. What does determine their sleep habits is temperature. They almost always fall asleep as the temperature begins to fall at night and wake up as the temperature rises in the morning. This habit suggests that humans may have evolved to sleep during the coldest hours of the day, perhaps as a way to conserve energy.

In the early 1990s, Dr. Thomas Wehr, at the National Institute for Mental Health, conducted an experiment to duplicate sleep patterns before the invention of gas or electric lights. He did this by placing volunteers in an environment lit with only natural light. After a while, his volunteers drifted into a pattern in which they slept for a few hours then awoke for a period of "meditative wakefulness" then fell back asleep again. Of course, we do live in environments of artificial stimuli—lots of it. But we adjust. As Dr. James J. McKenna, an anthropologist who studies sleep, says, "Our bodies move toward adaptation, not pathology. Given the sensory context [the stimuli of modern life] our sleep is probably appropriate to the challenge."

Yet, we're told that if we don't sleep eight hours, we're killing ourselves. Actually, just the opposite is true. Studies have shown that people who sleep between 6 and 7 hours live the longest. More than seven hours of sleep is associated with progressively increasing risk of death, especially from heart disease. Men who sleep more than eight hours a night have been found to have twice the risk of death and about three times the risk of dying of heart disease as those who sleep less.

Still, we worry about sleeplessness and look for remedies; exactly what the drug companies encourage. In 1990, five pharmaceutical companies established a National Sleep Foundation that labeled sleeping problems as "public health crisis" and a "national emergency." The sponsors of this so-called non-profit organization all manufacture sleeping pills. Their campaigns were wildly successful: between 2001 and 2005 sleeping pill prescriptions grew by 55 percent, to 45.5 million; by 2011, the number was 60 million. By 2012, four percent of our population was taking sleeping pills.

But here's the thing: sleeping pills, such as Ambien and Lunesta, aren't even especially helpful. In a 2007 study financed by the National Institutes of Health, these "hypnotics" reduced the average time to fall asleep by 12.8 minutes and increased total sleep time by only 11.4 minutes. One drug, Sonata, did not extend sleeping time at all. Test subjects slept six hours and 20 minutes whether they had taken a sleeping pill or a placebo. Such a paltry benefit doesn't begin to compensate for the dangers of sleeping pills—which are considerable. A 2012 study reported in the *British Medical Journal* compared medical records of 10,529 people who used hypnotic drugs with 23,671 who used none during the same period. They found that patients taking the sleeping pills on a regular basis were nearly five times as likely as non-users to die over a period of two and a half years. They also found that heavy users were more likely to develop cancer. Previous studies performed in Norway, Canada, and Sweden had also found a link between sleeping pills and increased risk of death. The Swedish study, which followed people for 20 years, found that regular users of hypnotics were 5.6 times as likely to die during the study period than those who did not use hypnotics.

It's normal for older people like me to sleep less than we did when we were young. Nevertheless, many old people turn to their doctors who prescribe sleeping pills, which are a class of medications called benzodiazepines (hypnotics). Joan Cook, a psychologist at Yale University, tells us that "Older patients are socialized to think their prescribers have some magic, a pill for everything." By taking such medications they face increased risk of falls, auto accidents, and reduced cognition. Some studies have suggested an association with

Alzheimer's disease. Dr. D.P. Devanand, director of geriatric psychiatry at Columbia University Medical Center, notes that "Even after one or two doses, you have impaired cognitive performance on memory and other neuropsychological tests." In fact, one study showed that for people over 65, the use of Ambien accounted for one E.R. visit in five. Nevertheless, the use of these medications continues to rise. In fact, among 65- to 80-year-old Americans, close to nine percent are using such drugs. Among older women, nearly 11 percent take them. Clearly, you're better off to trust your body to get the sleep it needs than to risk the side effects of sleeping pills.

Some researchers have found that many people, like me and the hunter-gatherer tribes, are natural "short sleepers" who average only 6.25 hours of sleep a night and suffer no ill effects. This group is healthy, optimistic, and has a high pain threshold. Being a short sleeper, they've found, is a genetic thing—a mutation, they call it—which has been shown to facilitate learning and memory, reduce anxiety and block the detection of pain.

Scientists understand the biological processes that tell our bodies when to sleep—our circadian system. But they don't understand the system that tells our bodies how much sleep we need. Not only that, they have also never figured out why we need to sleep at all. As one scientist said, "when it comes to what sleep is, how much you need and what it's for, we know almost nothing." So don't go telling me how much sleep I need.

16. On Your Own

I usually try to solve health problems on my own. When I'm stumped, I'll go to a doctor. More often than not, I leave the office frustrated, usually because he or she is unable—or unwilling to take the time—to figure out the cause of my problem. For example, I went to an orthopedic doctor because of pain on the side of my knee. Without missing a beat, he said it was because my knee "wobbles." He didn't ask any questions or look at my gait or posture. Later, I figured it out for myself: the pain is from an irritated sciatic nerve (your sciatic nerve takes off from your vertebra, then goes down your butt and the outside of your leg to your ankle).

One of the problems with doctor visits today—as I'm sure you've experienced—is that, because of the insurance reimbursement requirements and/or strictures imposed by their medical institutions, doctors are limited to fifteen minutes per patient and sometimes less. I try to be sympathetic with their plight. Still, it makes me mad. In their rush to move on to the next patients, doctors often fail to listen to and consider everything a patient has to say.

A 1999 study of 29 family physician practices found that doctors let patients speak for only 23 seconds before redirecting them. In the study, only one in four patients got to finish his or her statement. Here's an example reported on the PBS News Hour: a woman with an acute sinus infection went to see an ear-nose-and-throat specialist who, she said, "…looked up my nose, said it was inflamed, told me to see the nurse for a prescription and was gone." When she started protesting the doctor's choice of medication, "He just cut me off totally," she said. "I've never been in and out from a visit faster."

My sister, who is two years older than I, had been having shortness of breath and made an appointment to see a pulmonary specialist. After a long wait, the doctor came in carrying a large folder. He sat facing away from my sister, opened the folder and paged through the material. My sister tried getting his attention by saying she had some questions. He responded by saying he couldn't answer questions until he'd read the material. When she tried again to ask a question, he told her she would need some tests and that he couldn't tell her anything until he saw the results. Before leaving the room, he told her that "Barbara" will make the arrangements with the hospital. After waiting for Barbara to show up, my sister left the exam room and searched the corridors for Barbara, finally locating her sitting behind a desk and gazing into a computer monitor. Again, my sister tried posing a question, to which Barbara—while continuing to type—replied, "I can't answer your questions. You'll see the doctor after the tests." My sister never had the tests.

Even if a doctor listens to what you have to say, they often ignore your words mostly, I suppose, because they are the experts and you are not. (I call that arrogance). Ignoring a patient can lead to misdiagnosis. In her memoir, *Smile*, Sarah Ruhl tells of her experience when she was pregnant with twins. At one point, she developed a terrible itch all over her body. When she called her doctor about it, she writes, "...he told me that sometimes pregnant women get itchy. It's normal he said." Not being satisfied with that response, she searched the Internet and discovered a condition called cholestasis of the liver, in which bile leaks into your bloodstream, poisons your blood, and causes a terrible itch. More important, it can kill your unborn babies. Being convinced that she had that disease, she visited a different doctor who assured her that she did not have the disease because, he said, it's very rare. To reassure her, he did a blood test. It came back positive for cholestasis of the liver.

Studies show that misdiagnosis occurs in 15 to 20 percent of all cases, and in half of these there is serious harm to the patient. Case in point: My husband was prescribed a steroid called budesonide for his colitis (not the ulcerative kind). A few days after taking the medicine he began to feel weak and the muscles in his arms and legs became painful. He could hardly move. Nevertheless, he didn't want to stop taking the medicine without consulting the gastroenterologist who had prescribed it. He couldn't reach her for several days, and in the meantime his symptoms worsened. She told him to stop taking the drug, but never indicated it was causing his problems. To try to figure out what was causing his ongoing symptoms he went to his GP, his gastroenterologist, a neurologist, and a rheumatologist. They all had different theories.

In the meantime, I scoured the Internet and came across an "adverse effects" website called "Drug Informer" that listed 374 FDA-reported cases of "budesonide-related pain in extremity." The symptoms listed were exactly like my husband's, and many of the cases required hospitalization. One was listed as "life threatening." Armed with his information, I accompanied my husband on his visit to the neurologist. In the examining room, I mentioned my idea that my husband's problem was caused by the drug. The neurologist would have none of it, partly, I think, because budesonide is a steroid, which shouldn't cause such symptoms, and partly because I'm just an old lady accompanying my husband on his doctor visit. What would I know? I call that arrogance.

As a follow-up to the office visits, my husband had a colonoscopy and a muscle biopsy. The results showed nothing. When I was sitting in the waiting room after the biopsy, the surgeon who performed the biopsy came by. I told her my theory about budesonide being the cause of my husband's ailment. She said, "It's the reason I don't take pills," and walked off. That's the closest I got to an acknowledgement. It took my husband a year to fully recover.

In addition to time constraints and failure to listen, doctors, like the rest of us, are prone to cognitive errors—

the cause of about 80 percent of misdiagnoses. Dr. Jerome Groopman tries to help doctors become aware of their thought processes when diagnosing a disease. For example, rather than looking broadly at a patient's history and symptoms, doctors often pursue a single path of investigation; or they may be overly influenced by a patient's characteristics, such as obesity; or they ignore or rationalize contradictory data to confirm their initial diagnosis. Dr. Groopman also notes that "...research shows most physicians already have in mind two or three diagnoses within minutes of meeting a patient, and that they tend to develop their hunches from very incomplete information." One of his examples includes a woman who was diagnosed with viral pneumonia. It turned out her problem was aspirin poisoning. She had mentioned that she'd been taking aspirin, but the doctor didn't ask how many she'd taken, even though her symptoms were a classic case.

Chronic ailments for which cures have not been found force people to seek treatments wherever they can find them. Dr. Terry Wahl, clinical professor of medicine at the University of Iowa Carver College of Medicine, was diagnosed with secondary progressive multiple sclerosis. She was confined to a wheelchair for four years. "It was clear:" she says, "eventually I would become bedridden by my disease. I wanted to forestall that fate as long as possible." She devised a treatment for herself that consists of a type of Paleo diet, a strengthening and stretching exercise program, and neuromuscular stimulation. She now pedals her bike to work each day. (The Paleo diet, according to her, is a hunter-gatherer type of diet, one that excludes foods—such as wheat and cheese—that appeared after the development of agriculture and dairying. She also excludes plants in the nightshade family, such as tomatoes and potatoes.)

In chronic cases like Doctor Wahl's, for which cures are unavailable, "...ordinary people have to effectively become their own doctors...." Those are the words of Ross Douthat, columnist for *The New York Times,* who has chronic Lyme disease. He woke up one morning with a red swelling near his left ear and went to a walk-in clinic where a young internist gave him a cursory examination and told him that the swelling was just a boil and nothing to worry about. But Douthat got sicker, with his whole body "going haywire." He continued seeing doctors and was tested for Lyme disease. The test came back negative, which he later learned is not uncommon for Lyme disease. Because Lyme disease was ruled out, he went to eleven doctors in ten weeks, including a cardiac specialist and a gastroenterologist. They performed multiple stool and urine tests as well as cranial and abdominal scans. A neurologist told him that he had some sort of peripheral neuropathy and recommended exercise and more hydration—or maybe drink Gatorade for the electrolytes.

"All their tests were negative," he says, "each visit ended with the same gentle suggestion that I consider psychological explanations." He was prescribed sleeping pills, antidepressants, and Xanax. The tipping point," Douthat writes, "was my session with the head of infectious diseases at a major hospital, an appointment that took six weeks to get and that lasted all of 15 minutes. He listened to an abbreviated version of my story, sighed and leaned backward in his chair. 'Look, we've done everything for you,' he said. 'If you had an infection, we'd catch it.'" (Arrogance again.)

By the time Douthat's disease was positively identified as Lyme, he'd tried a variety of treatments, most of which were antibiotics of various sorts and various dosages. But the disease resisted every treatment he tried—those prescribed by doctors and those he found on the Internet, where, he writes, "...the chronically ill end up seeking out so many fringe ideas and treatments, trying out so many strange theories...doing science on themselves." It's what he calls "...home-brew versions of the scientific method." He believes that the doctor who finally diagnosed him with Lyme disease saved his life. But he also says he saved his own life "...because I was the only one who could actually tell what treatments made a difference. So I had to act like a doctor or researcher myself, reading online for ideas and theories about drugs and supplements, mixing and matching to gauge my body's reaction to different combinations."

I think this "home-brew version of the scientific method" is what you do when you've gotten no help from the professionals and have nowhere else to turn. You're more familiar with your body than anyone else. Not only that, but, like Douthat, you can also try different things to see how they work, then make adjustments. Of course, I'd draw the line at the truly nutty ideas, such as drinking bleach to cure Covid. I suspect that people with long haul

Covid disease will be in the same position as Ross Douthat, that is, having to become their own doctors and working out their own "home brews."

Friends and family can also be useful resources. Dr. Lisa Sanders, who writes for *The New York Times,* tells the story of a man who had terrible pain in his head, scalp, and jaw. A dentist told him it was TMJ—temporomandibular joint pain. "Lots of people have it," he told them. The diagnosis didn't seem right. The man's wife happened to mention her husband's symptoms to a friend, the director of an art gallery. The friend thought it was probably giant cell arteritis—an inflammation of the arteries in the brain. It was the correct diagnosis.

Another example of getting help from friends: I had plantar fasciitis (self-diagnosed). A guy in my exercise class said he'd cured his by taping the bottom of his foot in a certain criss-cross fashion. I found the instructions in the Runners World website and followed them. It worked like a charm.

As you know, the Internet can be an excellent resource, especially for those with intractable problems. One site, called Patients Like Me, is particularly impressive. It was started in 2004 by Jamie and Ben Heywood when their brother was diagnosed with ALS. Today, it's a growing community of more than 830,000 people with over 2,900 conditions who share their personal stories and information about their health, symptoms, and treatments. Another useful website is called Stuff That Works, described as "crowdsourcing treatments that work."

When you do visit a doctor, the visits should be collaborative: you and the doctor work together to figure out the cause of your problem. One medical model that takes this approach is called Functional Medicine. According to the Institute for Functional Medicine website, "Functional Medicine determines how and why illness occurs and restores health by addressing the root causes of disease for each individual." Its practitioners believe that "...prevalent health issues are mostly caused by the interactions between genetics, lifestyle choices, and environmental exposures and that treating them requires understanding these interactions and subsequently using that understanding to design appropriate treatments that are personalized to each individual." That certainly sounds sensible, but of course the treatment takes time and can be expensive because practitioners perform lots of tests. Moreover, your insurance may or may not pay for your treatment and, like doctors everywhere, the practitioners may vary in their competence. Still, if you have intractable health problems, it might be worth looking into. I Googled "functional medicine" and was surprised to discover that a medical conglomerate in my area advertises it: "Functional medicine doctors in the Sutter Health network partner with you to explore the root causes of your illness and create a personalized plan to treat your mind, body and spirit." Sounds good anyway.

17. Final Word

In college and graduate school, I majored in science. My life-long interest in the workings of the human body has kept me attuned to news and research about human health and medicine, some of which I question—such as the idea that you must drink eight glasses of water a day or sleep for eight hours at night. In those cases, I dig into additional research findings to look for more information or opposing views. The topics in this book reflect the results of that research. Incidentally, it typically takes ten years for the medical community to abandon a practice that has been found to be useless or harmful. Pity the poor folks who gave up eating eggs for fear of raising their cholesterol (eggs do not raise cholesterol).

As to my own health practices, I generally trust my body to keep things right—it's something our bodies continually try to do. For example, we maintain an internal temperature of around 98.6 degrees no matter the outside temperature. Our bodies can also maintain an acid/alkali balance as well as appropriate levels of fluid, glucose, and calcium. Our brains manage our bodies' levels of water, salt, and glucose. When we spend these resources by exercising, for example, our bodies respond by initiating an appropriate response, making us thirsty or hungry.

Even though your body does its best to keep you well, things go wrong. When that happens to me, I usually try to figure it out for myself. But sometimes I seek medical help. Example: I was wakened from a sound sleep because my heart was pounding. I waited for it to stop. When it didn't, my husband drove me to the emergency room, a 35-minute trip. By the time we got there, the pounding had stopped. Nevertheless, I had an electrocardiogram (EKG)—the test that uses electrode patches on various places on your skin to test your heart rhythm, blood flow, and whatnot. The results showed that my heart was fine. I was told that my problem was heart palpitations. Heart palpitations! I thought that was what Victorian women had when overcome with emotions. Like the vapors. I asked the doctor for further explanations. He said, "Oh, some people just have these."

In doing follow-up research, I learned that heart palpitations are caused by surges in adrenaline that affect your heart's electric impulses. You might get these from coffee or stress. In fact, I'd been having mild palpitations off and on when lying down, such as on the couch to read or on the floor in yoga class—certainly not stressful situations. I felt embarrassed at having gone to the emergency room for heart palpitations. On the other hand, now I know not to be concerned about these episodes—

should I ever have more. Oddly, I don't get them anymore. Maybe the last one jiggered the reset button on my heart.

About every ten years or so I get a cold. Because I've never been able to trace my cold to someone who could have passed it on, and because my husband has never caught a cold from me, I have a theory about it: I think I harbor a small population of the virus in my body and every now and then the population explodes. I've never heard this theory before, but, using the common sense I trust, I'm sticking to it.

Even though I don't have annual checkups or take prescription medicines, I do follow several standard health-related practices, such as exercise and eating a low carb diet (not a terribly strict one). I also believe in deep breathing. (Breathe slowly in, expanding your belly, to the count of five. Pause, then slowly breathe out to the count of six. Always breathe through your nose!) Deep breathing, or "controlled" breathing, is beneficial in lots of ways, including reducing stress, increasing alertness, and boosting your immune system. The practice sends signals to your brain that all is well, and your brain adjusts your parasympathetic nervous system—the system that controls unconscious processes such as heart rate and digestion as well as your body's stress response. Plenty of scientific studies support the benefits of slow deep breathing. By testing people's saliva following controlled breathing exercises researchers have found significantly lower levels of chemicals associated with inflammation and stress. Similar studies have shown that singing for an hour produces the same results. By the way, I only do the deep breathing if a situation calls for it—or in yoga class. I should probably do it more often.

Here's another regimen for healing: laughter. You might not be old enough to remember Norman Cousins (1915-1990). He was a journalist, professor at UCLA, and author of many books, including *Anatomy of an Illness as Perceived by the Patient: Reflections on Healing*. In 1964 he was diagnosed with ankylosing spondylitis, a degenerative disease causing the breakdown of collagen. He was in constant pain and given the prognosis of only a few months to live. As a professor, he had conducted research on the biochemistry of human emotions, which he believed were the keys to success in resisting and fighting illness. He decided to fight his disease with laughter (along with lots of vitamin C). For his laughter program, he'd watch the TV show Candid Camera and comic movies. "I made the joyous discovery that ten minutes of genuine belly laughter had an anesthetic effect and would give me at least two hours of pain-free sleep," he reported. He lived for 25 more years.

Laughter has since become a legitimate field of study (called gelotology). A related field, psychoneuroimmunology, examines the complex interactions between the nervous and immune system. It is now well documented that human emotions interact with the mind and body in complex and powerful ways that impact our health. As far as laughter goes, it profoundly affects a number of physiological processes, including decreasing stress hormones; increasing blood flow; increasing endorphins, the body's natural painkillers; and increasing the production of antibodies, which are important constituents of the immune system.

Stress can wreak havoc on your body in a variety of ways. When I was young, I used to get a rash on my chest whenever I was stressed. It was a handy way of letting me know I needed to chill. Dr. Bernd Heinrich in his book *Racing the Clock: Running Across a Lifetime*, speaks of getting mysterious joint pains that occurred during a period of "intense frustration." After achieving a breakthrough in his research, "the pain soon stopped as if I had simply turned it off." Stress is a physiological response to a *stressor*, such as a work deadline or scary medical test. It releases adrenaline and cortisol to help our brains and bodies deal with upsetting situations. In prehistoric times it was a useful response to a threat, such as a nearby predator. Today it stimulates the same behavioral response, but if the stress becomes chronic, your body stays in this fight-or-flight mode continuously, making you more prone to health problems, such as digestive issues, heart disease, and a weakening of the immune system.

Overall, I'm not much of a worrier. It feels like a genetic thing. I've never had a flu shot. The last time I had the flu I was in my 20s, so I don't worry about getting it. I also never worried about getting sick from Covid. Even though I take the pandemic seriously and got my shots as soon as they were available, I just couldn't make myself worry about catching the disease. Worry won't protect me. My lack of fear about it seems hard-wired. I can't help it. I decided to find out if there was a genetic component to fear and worry. It turns out there is.

Researchers have developed lines of mice in which all members are fearful. A newborn mouse from a fearful line who is reared by a fearless stepmother will still be fearful as an adult. Studies of adopted children as well as identical and fraternal twins reared either together or apart have also shown that fearfulness has a clear genetic component. Multiple genes and multiple processes are involved in fearful responses. For one thing, if you lack functional nerve cell receptors for a certain chemical (gamma-amino butyric acid), you will be more fearful. That's because the higher regions of our brains use the chemical to tone down our lower brain's initial impulses, which could result in an overly fearful response to stimuli. (The "lower brain" is the amygdala and is involved in fight or flight impulses.) Genes also affect our bodies' uses of serotonin, which regulates anxiety, as well as stress hormones. Maybe those genes explain my worry-less nature.

You may have health conditions that are a cause for worry. But you can reduce your worry load by trusting your body to keep itself in balance and ignoring advice to fix things that aren't broken—a practice that has worked for me. You can also try laughing.

Appendix: The FODMAP LIST

FODMAP stands for fermentable oligo-, di-, monosaccharides, and polyols. These are a short-chain carbohydrates found in many common foods. The FODMAP theory states that, for some people, eating foods high in FODMAPs causes an increased level of liquid and gas in the small and large intestine, causing symptoms such as abdominal pain, gas, and bloating, and sometimes diarrhea and constipation. If you have such problems, you might want to consult this list.

HIGH FODMAP FOODS

Fruit
Apples
Apricots
Blackberries
Cherries
Grapefruit
Mango
Nectarines
Peaches
Pears
Plums and prunes
Pomegranates
Watermelon
High concentration
 of fructose from
 canned fruit, dried
 fruit, or fruit juice

Grains
Barley
Couscous
Farro
Rye
Semolina
Wheat

Lactose-Containing Foods
Buttermilk
Cream
Custard
Ice cream
Margarine
Milk (cow, goat, sheep)
Soft cheese, including cottage cheese and ricotta
Yogurt (regular and Greek)

Dairy Substitutes
Oat milk (although a 1/8 serving is considered low-FODMAP)
Soy milk (U.S.)

Legumes
Baked beans
Black-eyed peas
Butter beans
Chickpeas
Lentils
Kidney beans
Lima beans
Soybeans
Split peas

Sweeteners
Agave
Fructose
High fructose corn syrup
Honey
Isomalt
Maltitol
Mannitol
Molasses
Sorbitol
Xylitol

Vegetables
Artichokes
Asparagus
Beets
Brussels sprouts
Cauliflower
Celery
Garlic
Leeks
Mushrooms
Okra
Onions
Peas
Scallions (white parts)

Shallots
Snow peas
Sugar snap peas

LOW FODMAP FOODS

Fruits
Avocado (limit 1/8 of whole)
Banana
Blueberry
Cantaloupe
Grapes
Honeydew melon
Kiwi
Lemon
Lime
Mandarin oranges
Olives
Orange
Papaya
Plantain
Pineapple
Raspberry
Rhubarb
Strawberry
Tangelo

Sweeteners
Artificial sweeteners that do not end in -ol
Brown sugar
Glucose
Maple syrup
Powdered sugar
Sugar (sucrose)

Dairy and Alternatives
Almond milk
Coconut milk (limit 1/2 cup)
Hemp milk
Rice milk
Butter
Certain cheeses, such as brie, camembert, mozzarella, Parmesan
Lactose-free products, such as lactose-free milk, ice cream, and yogurt

Vegetables
Arugula (rocket lettuce)
Bamboo shoots
Bell peppers

Broccoli
Bok choy
Carrots
Celery root
Collard greens
Common cabbage
Corn (half a cob)
Eggplant
Endive
Fennel
Green beans
Kale
Lettuce
Parsley
Parsnip
Potato
Radicchio
Scallions (green parts only)
Spinach, baby
Squash
Sweet potato
Swiss chard
Tomato
Turnip
Water chestnut
Zucchini

Grains
Amaranth

Brown rice
Bulgur wheat (limit to 1/4 cup cooked)
Oats
Gluten-free products
Quinoa
Spelt products

Nuts
Almonds (limit 10)
Brazil nuts
Hazelnuts (limit 10)
Macadamia nuts
Peanuts
Pecan
Pine nuts
Walnuts

Seeds
Caraway
Chia
Pumpkin
Sesame
Sunflower

Protein Sources
Beef
Chicken
Eggs
Fish

Lamb
Pork
Shellfish
Tofu and tempeh
Turkey

Acknowledgement

Many thanks to my sister, Elaine Greensmith Jordan, and my friend, Betsy Wootten, for their skilled editing of my manuscript. I am indebted.

About the Author

Connie Leas is an award-winning technical writer, now retired, and author of *The Art of Thank You* (Beyond Words/Atria, 2002), *Fat: It's Not What You Think* (Prometheus Books, 2008) and *Your Hands: How They Shape and Reveal Your Nature* (Mill City Press, 2013). She lives with her husband, Speed, in Boulder Creek, California.

Made in the USA
Las Vegas, NV
26 October 2022

58208809R00090